MW01088492

BUT I DON'T SELL

AN EYE CARE PROFESSIONAL'S GUIDE TO ~~SELLING~~ BEING MORE PERSUASIVE, INFLUENTIAL AND SUCCESSFUL

STEVE VARGO, OD, MBA

Steve Vargo, OD, MBA

Optometric Practice Management Consultant

IDOC

© 2018 by Dr. Steve Vargo

All rights reserved.

No part of this book may be reproduced in any form by any means without the expressed permission of the author. This includes reprints, excerpts, photocopying, recording, or any future means of reproducing text. If you would like to do any of the above, please seek permission first by contacting me at Svargo@idoc.net.

Contents

Introduction

"Selling is a natural skill. It's developed as a child.
You may know it as persuasion."
~ Jeffrey Gitomer

Selling. This is a word that sometimes elicits a negative reaction from health care providers. Somewhere along the way the word selling got a bad rap, probably for valid reasons. So, allow me to be clear from the beginning. At no point in this book am I suggesting anything that involves manipulatively twisting somebody's arm to make a purchase they do not want or need. In fact, this entire book is very pro-patient. Much of the content in this book came from my own frustrations with recommending or prescribing solutions to patients that I felt were in their best interest, only to have them decline my professional advice. "I'll come back when I have more time." "That sounds expensive." "Do I really need that?" "I'll think about it." Over time, I began thinking there must be a more effective way to persuade people. That's when it occurred to me, becoming better at selling required becoming more persuasive. If you don't like the word selling, then substitute persuasion. That's what this book is about – being more persuasive!

This book is not just about selling eyewear, it's about selling YOU. It's about creating an environment where people want to do business with you. It's about building trust and overcoming objections. It's about getting people to want to purchase from you, even when surrounded by less expensive alternatives. In terms of selling, this book is probably just an extension of things you are already doing. You probably have a website. Perhaps you have a Facebook page. You likely do some additional marketing, both internally and externally. And hopefully you strive to create a great experience for your patients, one worthy of their highest recommendations. Guess what! You're already selling if you're doing these things! Perhaps without even realizing it, you're trying to sell people on why they should come to you and not the competition for their eye care needs. Unfortunately, the problem I see with many practices is that these well-intended efforts are not enough. Patients are increasingly saying "no" to the independent practitioner, leaving doctors scratching their heads as the patient walks out the door with their script.

A study reported by Harvard Business Review that analyzed the behaviors of 800 people on sales calls found that only 37% of the salespeople were consistently effective, and of the remaining 63% many of their behaviors actually drove down performance.[1] That means the majority of participants in this study actually did things that *reduced* the likelihood of a sale. And these are trained salespeople! In comparison, how much sales training is the average employee provided in a typical optometry practice? Optometric training tends to focus on the technical aspects of the job such as operating diagnostic equipment, submitting insurance claims and performing frame adjustments. But sales training? Often times there is none, at least not at a level required to competently drive results. And if there is sales training, is it effective? Research published by both ES Research Group and CEB has identified that 85 to 90 percent of all sales training is ineffective.[1] This does not negate the need for training, but it does highlight that there is something horribly wrong with the modern-day approach to sales training. When you consider that most sales training programs conflict with the science of how people make purchase decisions, it's no surprise that the majority of behaviors salespeople engage in drive down performance. In the following chapters, this book will stress not only the need for more sales training, but also provide a framework for providing this training.

Would you do business with yourself?

As you will see throughout this book, I reviewed a lot of research on consumer psychology and what factors motivate a sale. My goal was to distill this research into actionable strategies that could be implemented by eye care professionals. In addition to researching the psychology behind why people buy, I also observed myself as a consumer. I would suggest to anyone reading this book that you spend the next few weeks or even months observing yourself as a consumer. This will likely be a very enlightening experience for you, as it was for me. Every day we are bombarded with marketing messages. TV and radio ads, billboards, social media marketing, salespeople trying to sell us something, etc. I read somewhere that the average consumer is exposed to approximately 10,000 marketing messages per day! The reality is that most of these messages we ignore. Many we don't even notice. We say "No" to the majority of people trying to sell us something. It's all background noise. But what about the ads that grab our attention? What about the salesperson that gets us to say "Yes!"? What was different about that situation or experience? Once you discover that, you can begin to implement these strategies into your own practice. It's likely that the same factors that got you to say "Yes" to an offer are the same factors that will improve sales in your own practice.

Let me stop here to pose a question, "Would you do business with yourself?" As you read through the chapters, you may ultimately discover that not only are you doing things that can drive down sales performance, but you might also come to the painful conclusion that you would hesitate to do business with yourself if you were the consumer.

What to expect

In this book, we'll cover many of the common mistakes salespeople make that drive down sales performance. As it turns out, if you want to be more effective at selling, you need to align your sales strategies with the way consumers process decisions. Much of becoming more persuasive with selling involves better understanding the mind of the consumer. Failure to do this often leads to, much like the salespeople referenced in the study above, a reduced likelihood of a sale.

This book will give you a framework for better understanding the psychology behind why people buy, asking better questions and knowing what to listen for, and addressing and overcoming common objections to a sale. We'll discuss how to get and hold people's attention with your message, and more effectively communicate the value of your recommendations. We'll present proven strategies for becoming more persuasive and influential in the minds of your patients, ultimately getting more people to say "Yes!" to you in an industry where it feels like more and more people are saying "No" to you.

In the end, selling is all about getting someone's attention and delivering a persuasive message. Now, if I have your attention, let's get started!

CHAPTER ONE:

The Role of Emotion in Sales

"When dealing with people, remember you are
not dealing with creatures of logic,
but creatures of emotion."
~ Dale Carnegie

P eople buy on emotion and rationalize their purchase decisions with logic.

You've probably heard this saying before. True to the saying, I'm sure most people can recall a time they made what's commonly referred to as an "impulse purchase." This could have been a chocolate eclair purchased during a point of low blood sugar, a pair of jeans that fit so well your credit card practically leaped out of your purse or wallet, or perhaps even a bigger ticket item like a motorcycle or Caribbean cruise. It's not that logic was not a part of the decision-making process; the point is that logic was not the part that initially got the buyer's attention – it was emotion! As a consumer, if you want to sell me something, you must first get my attention! The keyword here is not "emotion" or "logic", the keyword is "first."

The old vs. new brain

When I first became interested in the topic of selling, I came across a gentleman named Patrick Renvoise. Patrick is the author of a book titled *Neuromarketing: Understanding the "Buy Buttons" in Your Consumer's Brains*. A lot of the sales books and strategies I had previously familiarized myself with focused on what the salesperson needed to do differently to improve his or her effectiveness, without fully considering the mindset of the buyer. This book, and many others that address the neuroscience behind consumer behavior, focused on how consumers think, act and respond when being sold to. Have you ever been exposed to a salesperson giving you a long list of reasons you should make a purchase, and the only voice you heard was the one in your head screaming "Get me out of here!"

As it turns out, that voice was probably not coming from the logical side of your brain, but rather the emotional side. As you may recall from neuroanatomy classes, the brain has different parts responsible for different thoughts, feelings and emotions. The outer part of the brain, also known as the outer cortex or neocortex, is responsible for our logical and rational thoughts. When attempting to sell someone a product or service, this is often the part of the brain we try to communicate with. Here are all the logical reasons you should buy this product. Unfortunately, neuroscientists have discovered that the thinking portion of the brain is not the one that triggers the decision yes or no.

Most of our purchase decisions are originated from a deeper, more primitive part of the brain. In the medical literature this part of the brain is often referred to as the reptilian brain, first brain or limbic system. For the purpose of this book, I'll refer to it as the "old brain." I mentioned in the introduction that if you want to sell me something you need to get my attention. Well, more specifically, if you want to sell me something you need to get my old brain's attention! It's this part of the brain that will ultimately send a message to the outer, logical part of the brain to indicate either yes or no.

This is the rationale behind the phrase, "People buy on emotion and rationalize with logic."

The (not so) smart shopper

So, you think you're a smart shopper? You do your research and homework before making a purchase or big decision. You collect and analyze data and information necessary to make a wise, informed decision. There is nothing impulsive with the decisions you make. Rather, you are very rational and logical in your approach.

Below is story told by a physician involving a patient he was attempting to reschedule for a follow-up exam. As you'll see, this particular patient was also very rational and logical.

> *I suggested two alternative dates, both in the coming month and just a few days apart from each other. The patient pulled out his appointment book and began consulting the calendar. The behavior that ensued, which was witnessed by several investigators, was remarkable. For the better part of a half-hour, the patient enumerated reasons for and against each of the two dates: previous engagements, proximity to other engagement, possible meteorological conditions, virtually anything that one could reasonably think about concerning a simple date. He was now walking us through a tiresome cost-benefit analysis, an endless outlining and fruitless comparison of options and possible consequences. It took enormous discipline to listen to all of this without pounding on the table and telling him to stop, but we finally did tell him, quietly, that he should come on the second of the alternative dates. His response was equally calm and prompt. He finally said, "That's fine." Back the appointment book went into his pocket, and then he was off.[2]*

In case you're wondering, this patient was not an engineer. (Sorry engineers, we love you but you drive us optometrists a little nuts sometimes). What's going on here is that this patient had suffered brain trauma that affected his ability to effectively use the part of the brain responsible for emotion (the old brain). Thus, he was forced to rely on the parts of his brain responsible for conscious, logical thinking (the new brain). This is not how the average person processes decisions! While many people credit themselves with being "smart shoppers," many of our decisions, both big and small, actually occur at a subconscious level. According to Harvard marketing professor and author Gerald Zaltman, ninety-five percent of our thoughts, emotions and learning occur without our conscious awareness. And he's not the only expert who thinks this way; the 95 percent rule is used by many neuroscientists to estimate subconscious brain activity.[17]

Mental heuristics

A heuristic is a mental shortcut that allows people to solve problems and make decisions quickly and efficiently. Heuristics allow us to make quick decisions without having to continuously go through an agonizingly extrapolated process as described above. While most of us strive to make rational decisions, our brains are subject to cognitive limitations. Given limited time and information we have available, we are forced to rely on these mental shortcuts. Think about it, what if you had to go through this deep, logical analysis of everything from what to wear to work today to what to order for lunch? Not only would we burn out from all this mental effort, but we would never get anything done! The human brain developed to be much more efficient than this.

It's not that the mental energy we invest into decisions is fruitless, that's not the case at all. The point is that many, if not most of our decision are driven less by conscious analyzation and more by subconscious heuristics. Heuristics operate below the level of consciousness – the old brain at work again! And because these mental constructs operate at a subconscious level, they are not analyzed the same way a thought or belief might be. As a result, heuristics tend to be very predictable – and even irrational at times. Well known behavioral economist Dan Ariely has coined the term "predictably irrational" to describe this phenomenon. Once you better understand what heuristics are and begin to sell in accordance with them, you will be more influential with selling. Why? Because instead of trying to make the buyer conform to your model of selling, your sales message will instead be aligned with how the brain constructs decisions.

Many of our decisions originate from a subconscious level in the old brain. If you want to be more effective with selling, you need to be able to talk directly to the old brain! But there's something you need to know about the old brain…

I don't trust you!

You see, the old brain has some serious trust issues. It's been lied to, cheated on, and likely had a bad breakup with another business over the past several weeks or months. There's something else I have to tell you that you may not like hearing.

Your patients don't trust you!

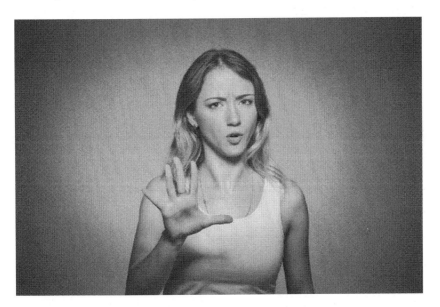

Oh, they know that you are a doctor. They see the letters behind your name and the degrees on the wall. All of this is very reassuring, from a clinical standpoint! They trust you as their doctor. They trust that the numbers you write down for an eyeglass prescription will allow them to see clearly. The patient with the red eye trusts that the eyedrop you prescribe will heal their eye. But guess what else they saw when they walked into your office? They noticed that you sell stuff. They glanced at a few of the price tags on the frames. Don't take it personally, it's not that they don't like you, it's just that this is our natural inclination as a consumer when someone is trying to sell us something. Figuratively or perhaps literally, we lean away, just as we do when a stranger approaches us on the street asking for money. The old brain, the emotional decision maker, is not comfortable in these situations. There's a trust gap that needs to be closed before the old brain will send the green light to the new brain to proceed. The question becomes how do we get people to go from leaning away to leaning in?

Common consumer fears

Let's look at some of the most common consumer fears:

- Distrust of salespeople
- Buyer's remorse
- Being lied to
- Incurring debt
- The unknown
- Bad past experiences
- Prejudice

Have you ever been given inaccurate or maybe even false information from someone attempting to sell you something? Have you ever regretted a purchase? Perhaps the item you purchased did not live up to expectations or didn't work as well as the advertisement made it appear. Does debt make you uneasy? Many Americans are in debt, but most would prefer not to be. What about the unknown? What if this doesn't work like they say it will? What if it doesn't solve my problem? Have you ever had a bad past experience with a company which forever tainted your perception of that company, or perhaps the industry as a whole? And what about prejudices? Has a patient ever expressed reservations about doing business with you because they read one bad online review or told you, "I heard you were expensive"?

What I'm describing above is not the exception, this is the mind of the average consumer that walks in your door. The same fears that you have as a consumer, your patients have as well. To the old brain, spending money feels risky, and the old brain HATES risk. Just accept this for now as we talk about ways to close this risk gap. However; if you fail to close the risk gap, these fears tend to become the very objections that prevent a sale.

Why do patients say YES to the doctor and NO to us?

I was recently talking with a group of opticians and one of them asked this very question. She mentioned that when patients are in the exam room with the doctor they are very agreeable to everything the doctor is saying. As the doctor goes through all the reasons the patient should have the recommended product or service, the patient affirmatively nods their head up and down in complete, or so we think, agreement. The optician continued to remark that once these patients enter the optical, they are no longer agreeable to the doctor's recommendations. In fact, she said that some patients immediately "shut us down." "I don't want any of that. Just give me what my insurance covers!" The optician was asking, "Why do patients say yes to the doctor and no to us?"

I'm going to suggest that this wasn't the case at all. Unless something really unusual happened in the hallway between the exam room and the optical that caused the patient to change his or her mind, I'm going to propose that the patient never actually said "Yes" to the doctor. More likely, the patient was just being polite and respectful with a series of affirmative head nods to indicate they were hearing what the doctor was saying. However; it's also very likely that the patient exited the exam room with one or more unaddressed objections, and this is what led to the patient declining the recommendations.

The opticians certainly have a role in sales as well, but if the doctor is sending a patient into the optical with unaddressed objections, this makes the optician's job very difficult. It might even prevent the patient from ever getting to the optical. A great way to NOT sell a pair of glasses is to make sure the patients never gets to the optical!

In the next chapter we'll look at the most common reasons people object to making a purchase and how to address these objections.

CHAPTER TWO:

Overcoming Common Objections

*"An objection is not a rejection,
it is simply a request for more information."*
~ Bo Bennett

In the book *The Science of Selling: Proven Strategies to Make Your Pitch, Influence Decisions and Close the Deal,* author David Hoffeld presents a series of common objections consumers have when making a purchase. He makes the case that these objections will cause the buyer's decision-making process to break down, which will in turn halt the advancement of the sale.[3] Below I will present the five most common objections I hear in eye care, asked in the form of questions. If you want to make more sales, you have to help the consumer overcome these objections.

Objection #1: Why Change?

Why do I need to change my prescription doc? I'm seeing well with the glasses I have now.

Why do I need prescription sunglasses? I've never had them before and I'm doing ok.

Why do I need to switch contact lenses? I know you keep recommending those daily disposable lenses, but I'm not having any problems with these 2-week disposables. I know that I wear them for a month, but I've never had the pink eye doc!

Recently a friend of mine mentioned that he was very disappointed with his most recent eye exam. When I asked why, he said the practice was very nice. A very professional setting with a large selection of frames. The staff was very friendly. They were a high-tech practice with a lot of impressive technology. And the doctor and staff provided me with a LOT of information, but…

"They never asked me about me!" he said.

My friend's dissatisfaction with his experience was because they provided him with a lot of information about eye wear products, lens technology and frame styles, but he said they never asked him about his profession, how he uses his vision, how much computer work he does or how often he's staring at his phone. There were no inquiries about hobbies or what he liked to do on the weekend. Ironically, a business that fixes eye problems never asked my friend about any eye problems *he* was having!

In sales, this is referred to as a "feature dump." This is where a long list of features or information is presented to a prospective buyer in the hope that somethings sticks. The problem with this approach is that it often does more harm than good. If nothing "sticks," then essentially you are giving this prospective buyer a long list of reasons to not make a purchase, upgrade, etc. In many cases you are making a great case for the buyer as to why they should NOT make a change.

Many people have what's called a "status quo bias." This involves a preference for the current state of affairs, and any change from the current state is perceived as risky. Obviously, a status quo bias does not bode well for getting people to change. The important thing to remember here is that for people to change, they need a reason to change that benefits them!

In later chapters we'll discuss how to structure questions that get people to open up about problems and concerns that motivate a sale. For now, just know that simply providing information is not enough. As I once heard someone say, "If information was all that we needed, we would all be millionaires with 6-pack abs!"

Objection #2: Why now?

What's the rush doc?

Can't this wait till next year?

I'll tell you what, just give me my script and I'll come back when I have more time!

In sales, it's generally accepted that the longer the sales cycle (the time between presenting a product or service and a purchase), the less likelihood of a sale. Recently a salesperson did a presentation for my wife and I at our home for a very pricey water purification system. She became a bit pushy at the end of her presentation and I told her that we would need to think about it before committing to a purchase. The salesperson then mumbled under her breath that no one ever calls her back after saying they need more time to "think about it." It was probably not the best sales strategy to mention this, but I believe that she was probably being truthful.

This has been demonstrated in eye care as well, as some studies have found that approximately 25 percent of patients who claim they will come back later to make a purchase never actually return, and the ones who do spend less money. In later chapters we will discuss how to deliver messages and sales presentations that "stick", but for now know that many of the things that you discuss and recommend to patients will be forgotten within 24 hours if not acted on.[14] Many of these patients who return several days, weeks or even months later have forgotten what you recommended and why you recommended it. "Oh yeah, I think I remember her saying something about that but I'm just going to go with what my insurance covers." When quality and value cease to be a dominant factor in a purchase, cost takes on greater significance.

There will not always be a justification for making a purchase now versus later, but many times there is. How often have you recommended or prescribed a solution to a patient that you felt was in their best interest and they resisted taking action, pushing off a decision until later? Are there times where you felt it was in the patient's best interest to take action sooner than later? This could be for clinical reasons or even a concern that if the patient did not follow your recommendations now, he or she may not take action at all. Some examples might be the early cataract patient who declines to purchase prescription sunglasses, the contact lens abuser who agrees to "consider" daily disposables at his next exam, or the convergent insufficient child whose parents want to "see how things go" this year in school before agreeing to vision therapy treatment.

While it's usually not the best course of action to make the consumer feel pressured into making a purchase (the "pushy" salesperson), are there times when building some urgency into your message will get patients to take action sooner than later? Nobody wants their arm twisted to make a purchase, but some people just need a nudge in the positive direction. When appropriate, help people understand why taking action now versus later is in their best interest.

Objection #3: Why you?

Why not the doctor across town? Why not the big box optical? Why not the Internet? Why YOU?

For this objection I'm going to lean on "trust." As a consumer, have you ever been in a situation where getting the best deal was your top priority? Of course you have! Some of this was a result of a knowledge gap. You lacked the knowledge and information necessary to make a decision based on value, so price became the most important factor. Perhaps this was a computer, car, health club membership, or even a new piece of equipment for your practice. But then something interesting happened. You conversed with somebody who started to fill in this knowledge gap. This may have been a representative or salesperson from the company. They asked questions. Became more familiar with your situation and how the product could benefit you based on your unique needs and interests. They also made you aware of what you would be losing by choosing the "cheapest" option. This person appeared to have a high level of knowledge with what they spoke about and your confidence and trust in this person increased. Based on this, you started to place more value on this person's recommendations. In fact, NOT doing business with this person began to feel… Risky!

2 ways to demonstrate trust

First, let me restate that the old brain HATES risk! It means well, as the brain has developed this safety mechanism to protect you from harm, including financial harm. However; risk can also be a major obstacle for people considering a purchase. Gaining someone's trust is critical to overcoming this obstacle. Trust quiets the old brain that would otherwise be yelling, "Get away!" In the mind of the consumer, the greater the trust, the less the risk. Let's look at two ways to establish trust.

- Demonstrate expertise. When we recognize someone as an expert we are more likely to comply with their recommendations.
- Communicate confidence. You need to do more than just present your products and services, you need to also display confidence. If you do not display confidence, the consumer's brain has a hard time placing confidence in you.[3]

As a licensed doctor, this may be less of an issue. You obviously have the expertise, and likely possess the ability to be confident in your recommendations. I think the same can be said of licensed opticians and anyone else among your staff with high-level training or professional certifications. But what about the rest of the staff? Trust can fall through the cracks in an office where expertise and confidence are not delivered on a consistent basis. This is often a staff training issue, or should I say "lack" of staff training. If you are able to gain trust in the exam room but send the patient to an optician or staff member who lacks expertise and confidence, the patient can quickly start having second thoughts about purchasing from you. Why? Because as trust wanes, risk elevates. Have you ever done business with someone who appeared to lack knowledge about the product they were selling and did not appear confident in their recommendations? How confident did you feel in purchasing from this individual? Perhaps you began having some of the thoughts below.

- I wonder if I really need these extra features?
- Maybe I should do more research before making a purchase? This person doesn't seem sure of what he is saying.
- I wonder if she gets a commission?
- This feels like a sales pitch!

Bottom line... doing business with people that lack knowledge and confidence (real or perceived) feels risky! Make sure you AND your staff are doing everything you can to make a purchase decision feel less risky. Demonstrating expertise and confidence is critical in gaining trust and closing the risk gap.

Objection #4: Why your product / service?

Many patients who walk into your practice have what's called a "commodity mindset." While we know that not all optometric products and services are created equally, does the average patient know this? There's a real lack of knowledge in the marketplace about the value components of eye care. There have been tremendous technological advancements in eye care. We have advanced diagnostic technology that allows earlier diagnosis of potentially blinding eye diseases. Pharmaceutical and surgical advancements in the treatment of eye disease allows for more successful outcomes with fewer side effects. Newer contact lens materials allow for fewer complications than previously seen, and technological advances in spectacle lenses allow for fewer complaints than seen with older materials. We are also seeing a trend in more optometrists treating more medical conditions and offering more specialized services that only optometrists are uniquely qualified to provide. Unfortunately, many uninformed patients lack this awareness and are unable to differentiate one doctor or product from another. When value is not communicated, price becomes the focus of a purchase.

In all fairness, it's not just patients. I've had doctors ask me, "How can we compete when we're all doing the same thing?" If that is your mindset and business philosophy, then I agree. It's very difficult to successful compete if you're "doing the same thing" as your competition. But before we throw in the towel, let's first explore some ways that you may indeed be able to establish a competitive advantage.

In business, there are two main ways to establish a competitive advantage:

- Be a cost leader
- Differentiate yourself from the competition

Being a cost leader is not easy. For most independent practitioners, it's not sustainable. As they say, there's always someone else willing to go out of business faster than you. But also take note that many companies that claim to be a cost leader are not successful with this strategy. By definition, there can only be one cost leader. Some companies execute this very well, for others it's a race to the bottom. Over the past several years we've seen many well-known brands go out of business. In the battle of price wars, there are few winners and many losers.

I think most private practice ODs reading this would agree with the sentiment above. While I do recommend having some budget lines and low-cost options to keep more sales in-house for the true price shopper, I think most would agree that trying to compete head on with the likes of big box opticals and online vendors is not a sustainable strategy. To the question of "How do we compete when we're all doing the same thing?", the answer is to STOP doing the same thing and differentiate!

Two rules for differentiation:

1. Must matter to the consumer
2. Must be unique

Many salespeople focus on what they think is most important to the consumer. This was the case with my friend I discussed earlier. They fed him a lot of information, but most if it was not relevant to him. If you want to differentiate yourself in the mind of the consumer, your message and presentation must matter to the person you are delivering it to. We'll go into greater detail on this when we discuss how to structure questions and use this information to deliver more impactful recommendations and sales presentations.

The second rule is to be unique. If you're still not sure what that means, let's peal back the layers to look beyond general eye care, eye glasses and contact lenses. Try to complete the following statement, "Many of our patients choose us because…"

Can you answer that question? If not, then give some thought to any reasons that your practice would be a superior option to your competition. This line of thinking must go beyond "glasses and contacts," and you really need to be able to deliver on your claims. Below I'll list a few unique ways to differentiate yourself.

- Legendary customer service
- Unique frame lines
- Largest frame selection
- Most technologically advanced office
- Specialized services (low vision, specialty contact lenses, vision therapy, etc.)
- Dry eye specialist
- Community involvement
- Convenient hours

Can you think of others? Perhaps your associate did a pediatrics residency, you have the most flexible return policies in your area or your practice does a lot of charitable work. Do some research on the local competition and learn about their offerings. What are their strengths and weaknesses? Once you have a clearer vision of your unique value proposition, then make sure that's not a secret! Build that into your marketing, branding, website and certainly your sales strategies!

The most important thing to remember as you balance cost vs. differentiation is that without differentiation, cost becomes the main factor for the consumer. Until you can complete the statement, "Many of our patients choose us because...", you will be forced to compete primarily on cost. Good luck!

Objection #5: Why spend the money?

As stated earlier, people buy on emotion and rationalize their purchase decisions with logic. Let's take a deeper look at that claim. What are the emotions that drive these purchase decisions? There are two dominant buying motives. These are the emotional reasons that people purchase.

1. Desire for gain. A positive outcome received after a purchase.
2. Fear of loss. Loss aversion is one of the psychological principles that heavily influences purchase decisions.[3]

One of the most common mistakes made by salespeople is telling the buyer what their dominant buying motives are as opposed to getting the buyer to tell them in their own words. This was the issue with my friend. The well-intended doctor and staff took the approach of telling him how he should spend his money without first uncovering his dominant buying motives – desire for gain and fear of loss. They made no attempt to discover the emotionally driven reasons that would motivate him to make a purchase.

One size does not fit all

I frequently hear both doctors and opticians complain about patients who do not accept their recommendations. Sometimes that involves not making any purchase at all. When I ask about their approach in presenting eye wear products to the patient, they almost always reply by telling me how they always recommend the best products and tell the patient why these are the best options. Not once has anyone replied to that question by telling me about the questions they ask the patient. This is a critical point. The information you provide is important, but it must be relevant. The key to becoming better at selling is not found in providing information, it's found in becoming a better listener! Rather than assuming someone's dominant buying motives, guide them in stating their own reasons and then use THEIR reasons to nudge them into a positive buying decision.

How do you discover someone's dominant buying motives? You ask! That's the focus of the next chapter.

CHAPTER THREE:

Asking Better Questions

"Successful people ask better questions,
and as a result, they get better answers."
~ Anthony Robbins

P eel back the layers, like an onion. That's how I would like you to think about questions. You have to peel back the layers to get to the emotionally driven reasons people make decisions. But not only that, this is how people naturally reveal information. In the first five minutes of meeting somebody, it's unlikely this person will tell you about the painful divorce he or she is going though. More likely they will tell you their name, where they are from, or what they do for a living. That makes for perfectly fine chit chat, but if you want to gain influence with people you need to go deeper. You need to get them to open up about their pain. You need them to tell you about their divorce!

Well, not necessarily the divorce (unless you're qualified to help with that), but we do need to know about the eye or health problems. We need to structure questions that get the patient to reveal deeper information than "I'm due for an exam" and "I ran out of contact lenses," but we also need to realize that not all questions are created equal.

Back to the onion analogy. Try to think of the onion like a brain. The outer layers of the onion are analogous with the outer layer or neocortex of the brain which is responsible for logical and rational thoughts. This is obviously a very important part of the brain, but not the lead decision maker. Remember what happened when our patient friend had to schedule a follow-up appointment relying solely on this part of the brain? We need to go deeper to get to the brain's true decision maker, the old brain. Questions are the tool we use to accomplish that. Peel back the layers!

3 layers of questions

Layer 1 – thoughts, facts and details

Below are some examples of Layer 1 questions. These questions are designed to gain a basic understanding about the patient.

How old are your glasses?

How often do you wear contact lenses?

Do you have sunglasses?

Tell me about any problems or concerns (yes, I realize this is not really a question)

Gathering thoughts, facts and details are very important. A doctor or medical professional must have a good understanding of this information to provide the best care. However; from the patient's standpoint there's no real emotional connection to this information. As you recall, we need to dig deeper with our questions to uncover the emotional reasons for making decisions. The questions above are engaging the logical, conscious part of the brain – the new brain. The old brain responsible for decision making is saying, "Wake me up when something interesting happens." If you want to be more persuasive with getting people to accept your recommendations, you need to connect your recommendations to their emotional motivators, not their logical ones. Peel back the layers!

Layer 2 – assessments and explanations

Layer 2 questions involve asking people to further assess and explain the information they provided from the Layer 1 questions. Below are a few examples.

Would you ever consider wearing contact lenses?

How does that problem affect you at work?

How did that condition impact your grandfather?

We've moved past basic thoughts, facts and details. We're not quite at the point where the patient is crying out, "Oh doctor, please help me! I'll do anything you ask!" but getting patients to open up about their emotional concerns regarding their vision and health is critical. I previously mentioned that if you want to be more persuasive with selling, you need to get the old brain's attention. Layer 2 questions allow us to say to the old brain, "Psst, you might want to pay attention to this."

The old brain doesn't obsess about facts and details. The old brain is very emotional, but the tradeoff is that it's not very intelligent. It struggles to process or make sense of words and abstract concepts. Medical information and clinical recommendations are not nearly as impactful without the old brain's involvement, and to get the old brain's attention your recommendations must be relevant. And I don't mean relevant to you! Sorry, but the old brain doesn't care about you. At all! It doesn't care how many years you trained to be a doctor, how much of a burden your student loan payments have been or whether or not your practice is successful. The old brain (yes, even the one in YOUR head) is very narcissistic. That being the case, appealing to its own self-interest is a very effective way to gain influence. What is the old brain most influenced by? Desire for gain and fear of loss!

Layer 3 – desire for gain, fear of loss

As you recall, desire for gain and fear of loss are the two dominant buying motives. That being the case, it only makes sense that asking better questions (the title of this chapter) should lead to the patient telling us their dominant buying motives in their own words. Below are a few example questions that get patients to reveal this information.

> *If we could treat your dry eye, how would that impact you at work?*

> *What impact would this condition have on your quality of life if it worsened?*

Ah, there it is! The old brain. Nice to meet you! Thanks for joining us. You know that problem you've been so concerned about? We were just having a chat about ways we could help you.

Examples please!

Ok. Let's do that. Occasionally when I lecture on this topic I'll involve a few audience members in role play. I ask them to be the patient and I provide some background on their problems and concerns. In one case I tell the audience member that he or she struggles with dry eyes on a computer, which is leading to a lot of problems at work. My job as their pretend doctor is to uncover those concerns (desire for gain, fear of loss) by asking a few simple questions. It usually plays out something like this:

> Doctor: Hello Mrs. Patient, how have you been?

> Patient: I've been great. Thanks for asking.

Doctor: Glad to hear that. Tell me about any problems you're having with your vision?

Patient: Well, I spend a lot of time working on a computer. That's what I do all day at my job. Everything is ok in the morning, but in the afternoon I start experiencing some dryness and irritation that worsens throughout the day. By the end of the work day I struggle to see my computer monitor clearly. I have to keep blinking to clear my vision. By the time I leave work my eyes are very red and sore. [Layer 1 information]

Doctor: Tell me a little more about how this impacts you at work.

Patient: For starters, I'm getting behind schedule at work with reports I'm expected to complete, and I've been making more mistakes which my boss has now brought to my attention on more than one occasion. Not to mention the annoyance of coworkers constantly asking me why my eyes are always red. I keep taking my contact lenses out to clean them, but that only gives me temporary relief. [Layer 2 information]

Doctor: If we could do some things that would allow you to see clearly throughout the day without all the irritation and redness, what impact would that have for you at work?

Patient: That would be great! I would be able to do my job much more efficiently and I'm sure my boss would appreciate that, along with making fewer mistakes. I might even enjoy work again! [Layer 3 information]

Let's do another example:

In this example, the patient has watched his grandfather gradually lose his vision over the years from macular degeneration. A once active and independent man, his grandfather now struggles with the challenges of vision loss. Even the simple joys of life such as traveling, sightseeing and spending time with grandchildren has been compromised. The patient doesn't express these concerns often, but internally he has a lot of anxiety about suffering the same fate as he gets older.

Doctor: Hello Mr. Patient. Please tell me about any problems or concerns you are having with your vision.

Patient: Something that has been on my mind is my grandfather. He's lost a lot of vision from macular degeneration. He can't do a lot of the things he used to be able to do. [Layer 1 information]

Doctor: That's unfortunate. Macular degeneration can be a devastating disease. Tell me a little more about your concerns.

Patient: It's hard to watch him go from an active and independent person to someone who needs to be constantly cared for. He has lost a lot of his independence. I have two sons and he's not able to enjoy time with his grandkids as much as he would like. Anyway, watching him got me thinking about my own future. I know macular degeneration can be hereditary and I'm worried that I may end up the same as my grandfather as I get older. [Layer 2 information]

Doctor: I understand. Your concerns are very normal. Given your family history, if we were able to do some things now that could potentially prevent you from suffering the same fate as your grandfather, would you be interested in taking those steps?

Patient: Yes, of course. I can't imagine losing my vision. I want to be able to play with my grandkids when I get older. [Layer 3 information]

The point of this exercise was to show the audience members how to get a patient to state their desire for gain and/or fear of loss in their own words. I wanted to demonstrate how this could be done rather quickly with a few simple questions. Who said this had to be difficult? Counselors and psychologists might have a lot of time throughout multiple therapy sessions to get patients to reveal emotional concerns, but many doctors and medical professionals work in busy practices where you don't have a lot of time to get this information. But if you want to be more influential and persuasive with patients, you absolutely need this information! Later we'll discuss how to tie your recommendations directly to the patient's dominant buying motives.

Does this information guarantee the patient will buy from you or accept your recommendations? No, it doesn't, but at least you have the patient's attention! Or should I say the old brain's attention. As mentioned earlier, every day we are exposed to thousands of marketing messages trying to sell us something, most of which we ignore. If you want to sell me something, you have to first get my attention!

Another key benefit of asking questions is that it directs the mind to focus on a single idea. Do you ever find yourself distracted with a lot of thoughts swirling around in your head? Job, kids, bills, etc. Guess what, your patients have their own issues as well. If I asked you what kind of car you drive, what would you immediately think about? You would think about your car. You didn't have to consciously tell your brain to think about your car, it did so automatically. That's the power of questions, it gets people to focus on what you need them to focus on at that time. The entire premise of selling involves getting people to contemplate your value proposition. To do that, sometimes you need to hijack the patient's thought process. Since you can really only focus on one idea at a time, it allows you to get the patient to at least temporarily suspend their thoughts on these other topics. Want proof? Try thinking about your car and what you ate for dinner last night at the EXACT same time. I'll wait. You can't do it, can you? Again, the strategy suggested above for presenting questions gets the patient to focus on what you need them to focus on. And most importantly, it guides the patient to the answers that solve their problems. This is why asking a distracted patient if they are having any problems with their vision often times fails to extract the level of information you need to persuade him or her to take a desired action. First you get the attention of the logical side of the brain, and then you dig down to the subconscious level.

Still not convinced of the subconscious brain's impact on decision making? Consider this. Brain studies suggest that we make decisions 7 seconds before we consciously become aware of why. Think about that. Research has found that subconscious activity precedes and determines conscious choice. According to John-Dylan Haynes, a Max Planck Institute neuro-scientist, "Your decisions are strongly prepared by brain activity. By the time consciousness kicks in, most of the work has already been done."[4]

Selling without engaging the subconscious, emotional part of the brain is the equivalent of trying to sell weight loss supplements using a lot of clinical and scientific information without using before and after pictures. Once again, good luck!

Paraphrase the patient's concerns

Value creation is not something you do *for* the patient, but rather *with* the patient.

Remember my friend who felt like the practice was focusing on what they thought was best for him, but failed to invite his thoughts? Let's try to avoid that. Using the examples above, once I'm clear on the patient's dominant buying motives, I'm going to repeat back to the patient what I heard and understood.

Mrs. Patient, what I'm hearing you say is that you are having a difficult time with dryness and irritation, which particularly affects you at work. You do a lot of computer work and your eyes become dry, irritated and red as the day goes on. Aside from physical discomfort, this is also negatively impacting your work performance, and you would like to be able to get through the day with clear, comfortable vision. Is that correct?

Paraphrasing the patient's problems and concerns back to them establishes two objectives. First, it lets the patient know you were listening and that you understand. Have you ever expressed your concerns to somebody only to have the proposed solution really miss the mark on what you were in need of? Were they even listening you wonder? If there was a misunderstanding, then this provides an opportunity for the patient to clarify. Back to the topic of risk, if the consumer suspects that the person they are doing business with does not fully understand their problems, then risk becomes a factor. As risk increases, trust declines. The consumer, or patient in our case, must trust that you understand their unique problems and that you are going to provide a satisfactory solution.

There's another benefit to paraphrasing the patient's problems and concerns back to them. Did you notice a word that I used numerous times throughout the example above? If it wasn't obvious, I'll use capital letters below.

Mrs. Patient, what I'm hearing YOU say is that YOU are having a difficult time with dryness and irritation, which particularly affects YOU at work. YOU do a lot of computer work and your eyes become dry, irritated and red as the day goes on. Aside from physical discomfort, this is also negatively impacting your work performance, and YOU would like to take some steps to avoid these problems and get through the day with clear, comfortable vision. Do I understand YOU correctly?

The word, obviously, is "You." The reason I sprinkle that word throughout the paraphrasing is because I want to give the patient mental ownership over the decision. I want the patient to feel like it's his or her decision.

I know some doctors and medical professionals will struggle with this one. I can hear some of you saying, "Who's the doctor here?" Others are proclaiming, "I know what's best for the patient and I'll decide for them!" Let me just say this, I completely understand the sentiment. Let me also say this, when it comes to human psychology, I don't make the rules! But here's what I can tell you, human beings are wired up to desire control over decisions and outcomes that affect them. Yes, even medical decisions!

If it helps, please be clear that I very much want the patient to follow my professional recommendations like any medical professional does. But also taking human psychology into consideration, people are more likely to agree and comply with things when they feel like they are involved in the decision-making process. My objective is to guide patients to the decision I want them to make, but if they feel like the decisions was theirs, or at least partly theirs, then I'm ok with that. When people perceive a decision as theirs, they are less likely to object.

CHAPTER FOUR:

Not All Problems Are Created Equal

"When solving problems, dig at the roots instead of just hacking at the leaves."
~ Anthony J. D'Angelo

O k Steve, fine, we understand that identifying problems is a good place to start when you have something to sell. But what about all the people that don't have any problems, at least not serious ones? In the last chapter you used examples of someone with chronic dry eyes and another with a family history of macular degeneration. Of course they are going to want help! But what about the patient who just wants a new pair of glasses or needs to update their contact lens prescription? The one who spends 37 seconds in our optical and then says they are going to get their glasses somewhere cheaper? And while you're writing up that glasses script, can I have my contact lens script also so I can buy them online? What about those patients?

Great question!

Let me first concede something, and then I'll ask you a question. I'll concede that not every patient has a significant problem that they are itching to resolve. Some patients just want an eye exam and a new pair of glasses which they don't intend to buy from you. But when it comes to identifying problems let me ask this, are you REALLY looking?

> Doctor: "Are you having any problems with your vision?"
>
> Patient: "Nope"
>
> Doctor: "Okee dokee"

You want to know a question I stopped asking years ago? I'll tell you anyway. It's the one you just read. "Are you having any problems with your vision?"

The majority of the time I would ask this the patient would say no. And then 15 minutes into the exam they are telling you about all the problems they are having. Or worse, you wouldn't find out until after the exam. You wrap up a contact lens evaluation, check the fit, do an over refraction, renew the script and send them on their way. Ten minutes later your tech knocks on the door to tell you that your last patient doesn't like the contact lenses she had last year and wants to try a different brand. Of course, the best time to share that information is at checkout!

So, my solution was this. I turned the question into what we might call a gentle command. Instead of asking, "Are you having any problems with your vision?", I rephrased the statement to, "Tell me about any problems you are having with your vision." Instead of letting the patient off the hook with an easy Yes or No reply, I forced them to at least ponder this for a moment. Try it. In most cases, the patient's immediate reaction will change. Instead of a dismissive shrug to indicate everything is fine, they actually stop to think about any problems they have been having. I found this to be a quick and effective way to get patients to reveal more information. Did they always have an answer? No. Was I able to extract more valuable information out of a greater number of patients? Yes!

This approach also takes into consideration that many patients with eye problems may not think they actually have eye problems. For the same reason patients sometimes say no to your question of whether or not they are experiencing any eye problems and later reveal problems they are having, patients sometimes perceive vision problems as normal or not significant enough to mention. Have you ever had a contact lens patient tell you they have been in the same brand for several years and they have never liked the contacts they were prescribed? Perhaps this was the reason the patient decided to switch doctors. When you ask if the patient mentioned this to their previous doctor, they say no.

The patient who initially says no to whether they are having any vision problems often sees their so-called problem as normal. Well, since you brought it up doc, my eyes do get uncomfortable at the end of the day with the contact lenses I have been wearing. But that's probably just dry eye, right doc? Oh yeah, my eyes also itch a lot this time of year. But that's probably just allergies, right doc? Pollen counts are high this time of year.

Thanks for sharing this info patient. And no, it's not normal. It's common, but it's not normal and I can help you with that. Would you like your eyes to *not* be dry and itchy?

Again, if you want to be persuasive with your recommendations, you need the patient to tell you about all their problems. However; as we'll discuss in the next section, not all problems are created equal.

Not all problems are created equal

Before you get too excited about a patient mentioning some infrequent contact lens discomfort or some mild glare with night time driving, we need to consider that not all problems elicit the same motivation to take action.

Let's consider two kinds of problems that motivate consumers to take action sooner than later. Below are three traits of people motivated to make a purchase.

- A need for the product or service
- The ability to pay for the product or service
- A sense of urgency about the decision

Let's assume since the patient is sitting in your exam chair or shopping your optical, they have a need for your products and/or services. While many people may initially balk at higher prices before value is established, most have the ability to pay either through private pay or through insurance benefits. The trait that motivates someone to make a purchase decision sooner than later is urgency.

Consider the corneal ulcer patient sitting in your waiting area crouched in the fetal position with his head in his hands wearing sunglasses. He looks miserable! This patient is not ready to hear about how excited you are about the new daily disposable that just hit the market. Maybe on a follow-up visit, but not now. Right now, he wants relief from the agony he is currently experiencing! That's the urgent matter that needs to be resolved.

Why do your contact lens patient come back to see you? Because you sent them a funny postcard in the mail with an owl saying, "I know whooo is due for an eye exam"? Ok, maybe some return because it's been twelve months even though they still have three months of unused contact lenses, but the majority return when they are running out of contact lenses. No more contact lenses raises the urgency to make an appointment with the eye doctor.

On this same topic, also realize that people are much more motivated to resolve internal frustrations as opposed to external problems. Consider the companies below:

- Dollar Shave Club
- Uber
- Amazon
- Netflix
- Warby Parker

These companies all operate in different industries, but what does each have in common? To rephrase the question, what does each one of these companies sell?

Each one of these companies sells convenience! They sell time! Me needing to get from point A to point B is an external problem. Me needing to call a cab, describe my destination, and then not know for sure when the cab will arrive is an internal frustration. Will it be five minutes? Twenty? I'm standing out here in the cold! Uber fixed that problem.

Me wanting to watch a movie I did not own was an external problem. Me having to drive to the video store, find parking, and then cross my fingers that the movie I wanted was in stock (the good movies rarely were) was an internal frustration. Netflix, and now a lot of other on-demand services, fixed that problem.

Curious what an external problem sounds like in eye care?

"Doc, I can't see clearly."

Blurred vision. That's an external problem.

"You can't see? Great! You came to the right place. We can help you with that! We sell glasses and contact lenses that help you see better."

"Glad to hear that," the patient replies. "But, can't I get glasses and contact lenses at other places? Maybe even cheaper? I'll tell you what doc, just give me the script and I'll think it over. Maybe I'll come back when I have more time."

Curious what an internal frustration sounds like in eye care?

"Ugh. Every time I try to hit a golf ball with these old no-line bifocals everything to the side appears distorted. I'm all over the place on the fairway and my putting game stinks!"

That's an internal frustration, similar to a patient who keeps making data entry errors at work or has trouble tracking a baseball or hates the way her eyes are red at the end of the day or had to stop driving at night due to glare. See the difference?

My point is that not all problems result in the same level of motivation to take action. Some problems are more tolerable than others. That doesn't mean as health care providers we overlook problems that do not register as urgent to the patient, but just know that good salespeople tend to be good listeners. Develop a keen ear for the problems that appear to be the most urgent and frustrating for the patient. These are the problems the patient wants to resolve now, not look around for a better deal or come back when they have more time. That's why I proposed the layer approach to asking questions. We have to get the patient to go deeper than "My glasses broke." I want to hear about how annoying it is when she plays softball and the glasses bounce around on her nose or how she hates the way she looks in glasses!" These are the problems the old brain is demanding a solution to. Build trust through your knowledge and confidence that you are uniquely qualified to resolve their pain and confidently guide the patient to a solution.

I'll think about it

And what about those problems that don't register as urgent or of high-level importance to the patient? As mentioned earlier, we never want to make someone feel pressured to commit to a purchase decision. This will come across as pushy and self-serving. It's not difficult to recognize when a salesperson is more focused on making a sale or earning a commission as opposed to helping us resolve a problem. However; are there times when a patient needs a "nudge" in the positive direction? This won't apply to every situation, but as health care professionals we've all experienced times where we felt it would be in the patient's best interest to act sooner than later. This could be for clinical reasons, such as the patient who foregoes your recommendation to purchase protective sunglasses or address their child's binocular vision disorder. As a professional, when you feel that a patient should address a problem sooner than later, then I think it's ok to "create" a sense of urgency. There's nothing disingenuous or unethical in giving a patient your honest professional opinion.

"I think I'll hold off on the sunglasses and get them next near," says the patient.

"That's an option, but please understand that your cataracts will continue to worsen at a faster rate without sun protection and I fear that another year without sunglasses could make it very difficult for you to do regular activities like drive at night and watch your grandson's baseball games. If your vision declines even a little there will be restrictions placed on your driver's license. I would strongly recommend getting prescription sunglasses at this time." The doctor replies.

Notice that we've also built desire for gain and fear of loss (dominant buying motives) into our case for making a purchase decision now.

Desire for gain: Continue to see at a level that allows you to function independently and continue to do activities you find enjoyable.

Fear of loss: Lose the ability to function independently and enjoy the same quality of life.

Would there be any problem with this patient returning in two weeks to make this purchase? No, there really wouldn't. But just keep in mind that many people who say they need to "think it over" or will come back when they have more time never actually return. The more time that passes between your recommendation and their decision lowers the level of urgency and importance for the consumer. In many cases, people forget what they were told and simply move on with their life. On that basis alone, I think it's ok to create some urgency merely out of concern that if the patient does not take action now, he or she may not take action at all.

In the end, it's the patient's decision, and they can still decide to say no. However; I'll sleep better at night knowing I strongly advised the decision that was best for the patient.

Tie features to dominant buying motives

Here's where your recommendations and prescriptions become more persuasive. Instead of just providing information, we can now craft a message that communicates directly with the true decision maker – the old brain!

So, go ahead and give the patient or consumer the information that they need. I never suggested NOT providing information, I just proposed that information a consumer does not find relevant will often prove to be surprisingly ineffective in motivating a sale. They will hear you saying the following:

We use state-of-the-art equipment to process digitally surfaced lenses. These lenses are custom made, designed specifically for your prescription. These lenses take into consideration eye dominance, how the eyes naturally move, head posture, and eye center of rotation. Digital technology allows both the front and back surfaces of the lenses to work in tandem to result in optically clear, distortion-free lenses.

This is all good information. Perhaps a bit overly technical for the average patient, but still solid information. Nothing wrong with educating and informing people, just understand that while your providing this information, the mind of the consumer is asking the following question:

What does this mean for me??

Aside from being a very boring presentation, information that is not deemed relevant to the consumer will fail to connect. Feature dumps and one-size-fits-all approaches to selling are rarely effective. In an era of limitless access to information, consumers don't lack for information, what they want is their problems solved. They want their needs met. They want their losses avoided. Stop being a walking brochure and start solving people's problems.

So, when you've taken the time to peel back the layers and uncover what people's real problems are, you can tie the aforementioned information directly to the consumer's dominant buying motives with one simple phrase, "What this means to you…"

What this means to you, is that when you hit a golf ball…

What this means to you, is that when you stare at a computer all day long…

What this means to you, is that when you drive at night…

All of a sudden this is no longer just information, it's a solution!

The stubborn mind

At this point you've peeled back the layers, got the patient to open up about vision problems and frustrations, and tied your recommendations and prescriptions directly to the patient's dominant buying motives. You've clearly communicated (when appropriate) why a change is necessary and why a change should occur sooner than later. You and your staff have established trust in the mind of the patient through your knowledge and confidence. You have differentiated yourself and the products and services you sell from the competition. So, this should guarantee that the consumer does business with you, right?

Unfortunately; not always.

I will propose that if you took the above approach you are likely much closer to a sale than if you hadn't. A "no way" might actually be a "maybe" at this point, but not quite a "yes."

As it turns out, the old brain can be stubborn. Even when presented with a solid case for making a purchase, the old brain can still have reservations. As a consumer, I'm sure there have been times when you thought to yourself, "This all makes sense and making this purchase feels like the right thing to do," but you just couldn't pull the trigger.

The trial close question

In sales they call it a sales presentation. For health care professionals, that term doesn't feel right. And frankly, this book really is not about sales presentations. It's about being more persuasive with getting patients and consumers to take positive actions. Selling glasses is certainly something that optometrists do, but we're also "selling" patients on why they should wear sunglasses outdoors, take their glaucoma medications, remove their contact lenses at night, and a host of other actions we ask of patients every day in practice. Instead of sales presentation, I'll just call it a "presentation."

Now that we've cleared that up, at the end of your presentation, I like to ask what's called a trial close question. It sounds like this:

What do you think about all this?

The reason I ask this is because the patient may still have questions, concerns or unaddressed objections. Again, putting yourself in the role of consumer, when you are considering a purchase but have lingering questions, concerns or objections, you're less likely to commit to the purchase. If it's something that you want or need, or something that potentially resolves a problem, then you're probably not saying "No" to the purchase, but you're not saying "Yes" either. You're stuck in a holding pattern with a nice solid "Maybe." And somebody better act quick, or that maybe will lead to you walking out the door saying you need time to think it over. And by the way, this is very much your old brain at play here. It's not holding up a stop sign in this case, but it is holding up a caution sign.

Back to the trial close question. If there are still any issues that need to be addressed before the consumer feels comfortable committing to a purchase, I want to hear about it. Asking the trial close question allows the patient an opportunity to express these concerns. People can object to a purchase for a variety of reasons. Maybe they don't fully understand what they heard. Maybe they leave for vacation tomorrow and can't wait several days for their new glasses to arrive. Maybe your receptionist made a rude comment and the patient decided to take their business elsewhere. All these concerns are valid, but let's spend a few minutes discussing what's likely the most common objection a consumer will still have at this point. The price objection!

The price objection

I mentioned that the two dominant buying motives for consumers are desire for gain and fear of loss. For some people, their dominant fear of loss involves losing money. The key to overcoming this is to establish a high level of value (desire for gain) in your presentation. When value outweighs cost concerns, people are more likely to make a purchase. From your own experience trying to convince people why they need the "best" eye care option, you probably realize this isn't always possible. There is a segment of the consumer market that can be categorized as true price shoppers. For price shoppers, saving money is a dominant motivator.

Below I'll suggest a 3-step process for dealing with a price objection.

1. Listen and empathize. At this point you've done everything you can to educate and inform the patient on the best eye care options for his or her specific needs. However; the patient has made the decision to not spend the money required to satisfy this need. The best approach is to listen and be understanding. Any sign of frustration or defensiveness will only result in the patient "leaning away."

It's likely the patient will interpret this as you looking out for your own financial interests while dismissing the patient's financial concerns. As a consumer, the minute you sense that a business is putting their interests above yours, there is a breakdown of trust. Remember, trust and risk are inversely correlated.

2. Repeat their concerns. "We want to provide the best eye care for all of our patients, but I do understand that cost can be a factor." Repeating the patient's concern back to them communicates empathy. Again, if consumers feel that a business is being dismissive of ANY of their concerns, trust begins to erode. If the consumer feels that the company is understanding and willing to address their concerns, then you might not have their business yet, but you still have their attention.

3. Reposition your argument. Once you understand the patient's concern and reassured the patient that you are understanding and empathetic, it's time to reposition your argument. Let's assume price truly is the major obstacle and the patient is not going to be swayed. Instead of watching the patient walk out the door with their script, use this opportunity to mention your budget lines. "I completely understand your concerns Ms. Smith. However; I do want to mention that we strive to meet all our patient's needs and we do have eye wear options for all

budgets. I may be biased, but I think we provide the best service in the area. We would love an opportunity to earn your business. Would you be willing to let our optician show you a few options within your price range?"

I can't promise you the patient will always say yes; however, I strongly believe that people want to do business with people they like and trust. Hopefully you're a very likeable and trustworthy doctor with a very likeable and trustworthy staff. Hopefully you've created a wonderful experience for that patient that leaves him or her wanting to give back. Later in this book we'll discuss the case for reciprocity and why this is such a powerful motivator, but for now just understand that when we like and trust a business we are more likely to want to do business with that person or company. Cost can still be an issue, but when price is the sole lingering obstacle, then remove the obstacle.

One final note on the price objection. This provides one final opportunity to restate desire for gain and fear of loss. "I understand your concerns Ms. Smith and we can certainly go with option B, but as a reminder that option will not provide the benefits we discussed, nor will it resolve the problems you were having with your vision."

Give the patient one last opportunity to mull this over. Nobody likes to lose things, and when the consumer hears about what they will be "losing" by not choosing your recommendation, the old brain is forced to ponder this before making a final decision.

I do understand that sometimes the objection is presented on the front end. For example, a patient sits down in the exam chair and immediately says, "I just want my exam today. I'm going to get my glasses somewhere else." When you hear this early in the process, just ignore it. I don't mean in a rude or dismissive manner, but just politely nod your head and continue with the exam. The patient does not have all the information yet to make an educated, informed decision. Go through the process suggested in this book and let's see if the patient still has objections at the end. It's better to deal with objections *after* all the relevant information has been presented. From your end, you can more directly address the specific objections as opposed to speculating why someone would not purchase from you.

To wrap this up and put a bow on it, you will absolutely not convince every patient to purchase from you. Sorry, that's just not going to happen. My goal for you is to minimize the number of people walking out your door with the intention of purchasing elsewhere. That, my friends, is a very realistic goal.

CHAPTER FIVE:

The Art of Persuasion

"Gentle persuasion succeeds where force fails."

~ Aesop

Research published by CEB, a leading advisory company, found that 53 percent of customer loyalty (customers choosing to buy from a company repeatedly) is not the result of the product, company, or service, but the behaviors salespeople use when selling.[3]

Let me repeat this – "the behaviors salespeople use when selling." There is undoubtedly an art to selling (or being persuasive) that goes beyond a standard sales presentation. There are certain behaviors that are critical to getting people to emotionally buy into what you are offering and then take action.

In this section I will focus on behaviors that have been scientifically proven to be very powerful tools for being more persuasive and influential. These tools are Commitment, Likeability and Reciprocity.

Persuasion Tool #1: Commitment

In the chapter on overcoming common objections, the purpose was to get the consumer to "commit" to doing business with you by answering the following questions:

- Why change?
- Why now?
- Why you?
- Why your products / services?
- Why spend the money?

Once the consumer has answers to these questions, it's much easier and less risky to commit to making a purchase decision. These answers are not obvious, and people in sales positions need to guide consumers in making a decision to purchase. When you cannot get a buyer to commit to the "Why" questions above, objections will linger which can halt the advancement of a sale. In fact, if further information or evidence is not presented, the consumer will likely remain committed to his or her objection.

The psychological principle behind commitments is that people desire to be consistent with their commitments.[5] I won't go into a lengthy political commentary here, but politics are a great example. Have you noticed that regardless of political affiliation, many people are willing to overlook a number of indiscretions and questionable decisions by politicians when the politician is the one they voted for?

Even amidst numerous scandals and improprieties, people are reluctant to publicly condemn or turn their back on their candidate of choice. After all, this is the candidate they committed to.

This is certainly not unique to politics. I mentioned in an earlier chapter that just because a patient appears to agree with a doctor's recommendations in the exam room by listening intently and nodding their head up and down does not necessarily mean the patient has committed to making a purchase or taking a desired action. Comprehension of an idea does not directly convert to action. Getting the patient or consumer to verbally *commit* to a desired action will more predictably influence their behaviors.

In the best-selling book *Influence: The Psychology of Persuasion* by Dr. Robert Cialdini, he devotes an entire chapter to the topic of commitment. Dr. Cialdini offers numerous examples of how our commitments can drive our actions and beliefs. For example, one study found that people at a racetrack were more confident of their horse's chances of winning immediately after they placed their bets. Another study found that when people were asked and agreed to collect donations for the American Cancer Society, there was a 700 percent increase in volunteers when a representative of the American Cancer Society called a few days later to ask for neighborhood canvassing. In yet another study, people were considerably more likely to intervene during a theft (in this study a theft was staged after a beach dweller walked away from her blanket) when the person was asked to "watch my things" as opposed to being a casual observer. 19 of 20 people who were asked to watch the person's belongings responded to the theft as opposed to only 4 of 20 who were not asked. According to Cialdini, "Once we make a choice or take a stand, we will encounter personal and interpersonal pressures to behave consistently with that commitment." In short, not being consistent with our commitments is perceived as a character weakness associated with dishonesty and unreliability.[5]

Many eye care practices struggle with patient no-shows. One of my favorite examples of how the principle of commitment can transform a business comes from a piece in the New York Times titled, "In War Against No-Shows, Restaurants Get Tougher." The article featured a popular restaurant in Chicago called Gordon's that was losing $900,000 a year because of its 30 percent no-show rate. Remarkably, the restaurant was able to drastically reduce its no-show rate with one simple change to the reservation process. In the past, when taking a reservation a Gordon's employee would say, "Please call us if you change your plans." With this approach, three out of every ten reservations resulted in a no-show. However, once the statement was changed to a question that inspired a commitment - "Will you call us if you change your plans?"- no-shows plummeted to 10 percent! The subtle shift was the receptionist's request for (and pause for) the caller's promise.[6]

Below are a few questions that can make your presentations more powerful by soliciting a commitment from the patient:

- Would you like to move forward?
- Are you ready to try contact lenses?
- When would you like to schedule your evaluation?
- Will you make sure to take your prescription eyedrops as prescribed?
- Knowing what you know now, would you ever sleep in your contact lenses again?
- Is there any reason you would purchase glasses without the features we discussed?
- Based on the current state of your cataracts, do you really want to postpone getting prescription sunglasses?

As mentioned, this book is not solely focused on "selling," it's about becoming more persuasive with getting people to take desirable actions that you feel are in their best interest. Getting people to verbally commit to these actions is very powerful. Remember, it's human nature to desire to be consistent with things we commit to. In fact, when we verbally commit to something it alters our own self-perception. Once we agree to donate to a charitable cause, we see ourselves as charitable and desire to act consistent with this self-perception. This is the reason that writing down and sharing your goals and publicly announcing your intention to join a gym and lose 20 pounds is more powerful than keeping this information to yourself. In fact, many weight loss clinics require people to immediately write down a weight loss goal and show that goal to as many friends, relatives and neighbors as possible. Not only is there now a commitment that we want to remain consistent to, but we also see ourselves in a different light as someone who is goal-oriented, health conscious, or whatever motive we have committed to achieving.

Commitments demand action, instructions and recommendations do not. And as discussed earlier, people like to be included in decisions that affect them. Getting someone to publicly commit to taking action transfers some ownership of the process over to them, where being told or instructed what to do in a one-way fashion is less effective with inspiring action.

What about a weak commitment? It would be great if a commitment always involved a patient leaping out of the exam chair and running into the optical yelling from the top of their lungs "Let's do this!", but not every commitment you'll hear is this enthusiastic.

Doctor: Will you promise me that you will stop sleeping in your contact lenses?

Patient: I'll do my best.

Hmm. Not very convincing, is it? A good way to address this is to revisit the topic of emotional motivators. If you sense that someone is not entirely committed to an idea, ask the patient a question that requires them to verbalize desire for gain or fear of loss.

Doctor: Your best, huh? Well that's a start, but if you slip back into your old ways how will you handle wearing glasses all the time if you continue to damage your eyes and can no longer safely wear contact lenses?

The patient now has to think through the value of taking this desired action while verbally stating the intrinsic motivators that support a commitment.

I made a promise

Put yourself in the position of someone whose child requested a specific toy for Christmas, whose fitness trainer suggested a specific diet, or whose boss mentioned completing a certain project. While there may be some sense of obligation on your part to comply with these requests, how would this sense of obligation change if you had committed to taking these actions? For those of you with kids, have you ever found yourself saying "I promised little Johnny I would buy it for him." And off to the store you went! I told my trainer I wouldn't eat junk food. I assured my boss this project would be completed by next Friday. This feels different, right? Not complying with these commitments just feels wrong!

Did you know that a common tactic used by toy manufac-turers is to heavily advertise a new toy months before

Christmas and then undersupply the stores?[5] Why would they do this? Parents, obligated with keeping little Johnny or Sally happy, will of course overcompensate for the lack of this year's hottest toy by purchasing numerous other toys for the kids to rip open on Christmas morning. And when the hot new toy reappears in the stores at the end of January, guess who treks back to the toy store with credit card in hand? Well, you know, I promised little Johnny I would buy it for him.

"I'll try, but if I can't get it for you now, I'll get it for you later." – a Hasbro spokesperson when asked what parents should say to their kids who wanted a toy in high demand and low supply.[5]

Start small

As it applies to optometry and being more persuasive, getting commitments is more effective when it's a series of small commitments that lead to bigger commitments. Too often people in sales positions fail to do this and try to close the deal at the end by asking the consumer to make one BIG commitment – purchase from you! Smaller commitments throughout the process help get your foot in the door, as they say. Some examples below:

- Do you agree with what I'm saying?
- Are you ok with what I'm suggesting?
- Are you open to trying this?

A fascinating study that exemplifies this was conducted by two social scientists in 1966. A researcher, posing as a volunteer worker, went door to door in a residential California neighborhood asking homeowners to allow a public-service billboard to be installed on their front lawns. To give the homeowner an idea of what the sign would look like, they were shown a photograph of a house which was almost completely obstructed by a very large sign reading DRIVE CAREFULLY. Not surprising, the majority of people declined. Only 17 percent complied. However, there was one particular group that responded quite favorably. In fact, 76 percent of them complied to the request.

The difference in responses traced back to something that took place two weeks earlier. In this group a different volunteer worker had come to their doors and asked them to display a three-inch square sign in a front window that read BE A SAFE DRIVER. Nearly everyone agreed to this "small commitment." Innocently complying with this rather small safe-driving request led to this group becoming remarkably willing to comply with a much bigger request when later asked to allow the billboard on their front lawn.[5] That's the power of commitment!

It's important to note that the tools of persuasion can be used for good or they can be used for evil (insert evil laugh). Even Dr. Cialdini acknowledges in his book that as a consumer or the recipient of a request, we should exercise caution to not get manipulated into taking an action that we do not want to or that is not in our best interest simply because we made a commitment. I'll use this opportunity to repeat that while I am sharing science and research that demonstrates ways to be more persuasive and influential, my intent for the reader is to use this information strictly for good.

The important takeaway: Smiles and polite head nods are not commitments. If you want to be more persuasive with getting patients to take action, you'll need to inspire them to make a commitment.

Persuasion Tool #2: Likeability

Think about somebody you are almost indifferent to. You neither like nor dislike this person. Now imagine this person offers you a friendly compliment, or a mutual friend mentioned that she said something very positive about you. It changes your perception about this person in a positive way, right?

Now put yourself in the position of a consumer. Are you more likely to buy from someone you are indifferent to or someone you genuinely like? A vast amount of research has shown that not only does likeability influence buying decisions, but likeability is a significant factor in someone's ability to influence another person.[3]

Years ago, a colleague of mine commented that the doctor she worked with produced at a much higher level than she did. Apparently, many of the patients that he saw purchased eye wear from their optical, where many of her patients requested their script to purchase elsewhere. In an offhanded and almost dismissive explanation of this, she claimed "people only buy from him because he's nice to them!"

When I asked her to expand on that, she said he had a very charismatic personality. He was very good at finding common interests with patients and always started off the exam with a friendly discussion. She would often times hear laughing coming from the room, and she also admitted he wasn't too hard on the eyes and was popular with the female patients. How dare he be so damn likeable!

In my previous book, *Eye on Leadership: An optometrist's game plan for creating a motivated and empowered team*, I discuss a lot of the qualities that influential people tend to have. I also do a lot of lecturing on the topic of leadership, and one of the more interesting studies that I've shared focuses on the positive outcome of likeability. A study published in *Harvard Business Review* analyzed the traits of 51,836 leaders. Guess how many of these nearly 52K leaders rated near the bottom on likeability and high on leadership effectiveness. Twenty-seven! Yes, that's a 2 followed by a 7. That means that the probability of a leader being disliked yet effective in a leadership role is about 1 in 2,000.[7]

While the dynamics are different in a selling scenario, the relationship still matters, even if it's a recently established relationship. I started off the book mentioning that nothing in this book involves anything manipulative or unethical. No arm twisting or shallow tricks. These things will make you come off as unethical and phony.

To state the obvious, if you're not a likeable person, you have a steep hill to climb when it comes to selling. Your ability to persuade and influence is severely diminished when people don't like you. Also keep in mind that reasons for disliking a person can be rather subtle. Perhaps the salesperson did not smile when she introduced herself, didn't show concern with the problem you were having, or made a comment that you interpreted as snide or condescending. Remember, the old brain makes fast and hasty decisions. It's not always rational, but it's often predictable. If someone doesn't like you, they are much less likely to want to do business with you. Consumers do not lean into unfriendly people, they lean away. In the world of selling, likeability is not a luxury, it is a prerequisite!

How to be more likeable

I started off this section discussing how we tend to like people who like us. Numerous studies have found that when we perceive that someone likes us, we look upon them more favorably.[8] If you want your patients and consumers to like you, show them that you like them. A straightforward way to do this is to mention something that you truly appreciate about the person. Some examples below. Before getting too personal with a compliment (ie. You look great in those jeans!), consider the appropriateness of your remarks. I think these are relatively safe.

- I appreciate you being so patient. I apologize for the wait!
- Your kids are very polite. You must be proud!
- I love your new hairstyle!
- I appreciate you not sleeping in your contact lenses as we discussed.
- Thank you for being a loyal patient.
- The staff always looks forward to you coming in.
- You're hilarious. You always make me laugh!
- Thank you for the referrals. We truly appreciate it!
- You're a very kind and caring person.

Again, this is not intended to be manipulative (am I beating a dead horse about that?). Find something you genuinely appreciate or admire about the other person and communicate it to that person. If you honestly can't think of anything to say, then don't say anything, but I think too often we hold back these comments because we fear it might be awkward to mention. Yet, who wouldn't like to hear any of the comments listed above?

Why do I like you?

Digging further into the science of likeability, Dr. Cialdini's research uncovered a number of factors that reliably cause liking.[5] And without realizing it, we have all likely said yes to the requests of others based on the following factors.

- Physical attractiveness. Research has shown that we automatically assign qualities such as talent, kindness, honesty and intelligence to good-looking people. This is often referred to as the halo effect. Furthermore, we do this without even realizing that physical attractiveness plays a role in these judgments.

- Similarity. If you're not blessed with the looks of a Hollywood actor or actress, don't fret. Similarity is one of the most influential factors in likeability. In the areas of opinions, personality traits, background, and lifestyle, we like people who are similar to us. Even seemingly trivial things like how someone dresses or what music they listen to can make someone appear more likeable if their preferences are aligned with ours. In one study where people were asked to rank-order a waiting list of patients suffering from kidney disorder to determine their deservedness for the next available treatment, people chose those whose political party preference matched their own. Several studies have even found that mirroring another person's verbal or nonverbal behaviors makes us more likeable.[3]

- Compliments. Human beings are phenomenal suckers for flattery. Although our gullibility has limits, especially when we sense that someone is providing a compliment in exchange for something – as a rule we tend to believe praise and like those who provide it. As discussed above, there are numerous ways to communicate to someone that you like and appreciate them.

The buyer's emotional state

Emotions play an integral role in how the brain processes decisions. Numerous scientific studies have shown that experiencing positive emotions enhances the mental capacity to make decisions and increases receptiveness to persuasive requests.[3] Ask yourself if you are more likely to make a purchase when feeling positive and optimistic. Conversely, when the brain is experiencing negative emotions, it struggles to perceive value and often rejects the ideas or suggestions that are in the person's best interest.

The patient's emotional state needs to be considered in these situations. If the patient appears to be in a sour mood, distracted or annoyed, there's a good chance this person is not in a buying mood, and they may not even be receptive to what you are saying. How do you alter this person's mood? Well, you could follow the direction of the doctor mentioned above and talk about things that stimulate good feelings. Published studies have confirmed that when sales situations begin with casual chitchat, a favorable outcome is more likely to occur.[9] Try smiling more. It's hard to stay in a bad mood when the person you're talking to keeps smiling! Talk about things that naturally stimulate positive feelings in most people like family, hobbies or vacations. I'm not suggesting you spend twenty minutes in trivial conversation with every patient (your staff will hate you!) but do take the temperature of your patient's mood on the front end to determine if you need to inject a little positivity into their day! Sending an irritable, distracted patient into the optical does not bode well for sales.

Persuasion Tool #3: Reciprocity

The law of reciprocity is one of the most powerful tools of influence around us. The rule essentially says that we should repay what another person has provided us. In fact, the social pressure to repay the other person is so strong that we feel *obligated* to repay the outstanding debt, even if the "debt" is nothing more than a small favor or gift – like a soft drink.

One of the more famous experiments examining reciprocity involved two subjects who were rating the quality of some paintings as part of an experiment on art appreciation. One of the subjects, we'll call him Tim, was only posing as a fellow subject and was actually an assistant of the psychologist conducting the experiment. The experiment took place under two different conditions. In some cases, Tim left the room for a two-minute break returning with two bottles of Coca-Cola, offering one to the other subject. In other cases, Tim returned empty-handed.

After all the paintings were rated, Tim then asked the other subject for a favor. He said he was selling raffle tickets for a new car and could win $50 if he sold the most tickets. Tim's request was for the subject to buy some raffle tickets at 25 cents each. Apparently feeling that they owed him for the earlier favor, the subjects who received the soft drink purchased twice as many tickets as the subjects who had not been given the earlier favor.[5] This is just one study of many that have consistently demonstrated the power of the law of reciprocity.

Any Seinfeld fans here? I realize this is fiction, but one particular episode that comes to mind was a great example of the law of reciprocity. In the episode, Jerry accepts an Armani suit from a fellow comedian named Kenny Bania. The suit is an unsolicited gift, and it's important to mention that Jerry is not at all fond of Kenny, to the point that he is reluctant to accept the gift fearing a favor will be asked in return. Sure enough, after a few moments of gloating over what a great gesture this was, Kenny offhandedly mentions that Jerry can return the favor by treating him to a meal. Jerry dislikes Kenny so much that he regrets ever accepting the gift, but now feels obligated to treat him to a meal at a fine restaurant. Even when Kenny mentions while seated at the table of the restaurant that he isn't hungry and will save the dinner for another time, Jerry still agrees to arrange another dinner to clear the debt.

I'm pretty sure I've exceeded my quota for mentioning the purpose of this book is not to manipulate, but there's no denying the power of this tool of influence. It creates a social obligation that at times is almost impossible to avoid. And circling back to the above referenced Seinfeld episode, have you ever found yourself in the position of Jerry?

My time is valuable!

Doctors often have a reluctance to give anything away for free. I am certainly sympathetic to the reasons, as many health care professionals are under the increasing pressure of declining 3rd party reimbursements along with a seemingly growing segment of the population that expects health care services to be provided at no cost. Why do I have a copay? Nobody told me about a deductible! Just give me what my insurance covers. Do I have to pay for this? Doctors often reply with a defensive stance of their own. If patients don't respect my time, they can go somewhere else!

Is there a balance here where doctors can give freely to patients without compromising their professional values and standards? Is there a point where altruistic generosity can supersede the devaluation of services? Below I would like to share a previous article I wrote on the topic of reciprocity titled "Optometry and the Law of Reciprocity: Does It Really Exist?"

Doctor: Would you like to order your contacts today, Mrs. Smith?

Mrs. Smith: That's OK. I'll just take the prescription and get them online.

What happened here? You just did a thorough, high-tech eye exam on Mrs. Smith, addressed all her complaints, answered all her questions, and then without hesitation she informs you that she will be taking her business elsewhere. Let's rewind 20 minutes and see if there's anything we could have done to elicit a different response.

In the book *Influence: The Psychology of Persuasion*, Robert Cialdini takes an insightful look at the power of persuasion and what causes people to say yes (or no) to what you are offering. According to Dr. Cialdini, one of the most potent weapons of influence is reciprocity. Reciprocity refers to responding to a positive action with another positive action. In other words, when somebody does something nice for us, we feel an obligation to return the gesture.

Some of the experiments involved offering someone a soft drink and then later asking the recipient to buy raffle tickets. The subjects who were offered the drink bought twice as many raffle tickets as the control subjects that were not offered a drink. In another experiment, tips increased significantly at a restaurant when the waitress left a complimentary mint with the bill. Tips increased even further when two mints were left.

Some "acts of kindness" we might offer our patients:

- Offer to clean and adjust glasses for people who are just browsing
- Gift box with free solution, cleaning towels, etc.
- In-office coupons or discounts
- Free brochures and literature
- Starbucks gift cards
- Free Wi-Fi
- Complimentary coffee
- Give eye related toys to the little ones
- Walk an elderly patient to his/her car

It's important to discern that while there is a strong cultural pressure to reciprocate a gift, there is no such pressure to purchase an unwanted commercial product. Although we give a great deal to our patients, if our presentation communicates standard operating procedure instead of selfless generosity, our patients will see it that way also. If our patients don't perceive our actions as altruistic, from a social behavioral standpoint there exists no perceived obligation on their part to reciprocate. I'm not suggesting anybody take this approach for strictly self-serving reasons. If you approach this with exploitative motives, your patients will likely see through the facade and turn away.

While the law of reciprocity can be exploited and used to manipulate, you probably won't find long-term success in that approach. As health care providers, we routinely give to our patients in a spirit of altruism for the same reason we became optometrists: we like to help others.

Is there anything wrong with giving with no expectation of receiving anything in return …and the recipient responds by giving back? I don't think so. I think this exchange appeals to the positive side of human nature. If you take this approach, maybe next time the previous exchange will go something like this:

> Doctor: Would you like to order your contacts today Mrs. Smith?
>
> Mrs. Smith: Sure. That would be great.

CHAPTER SIX:

Less is More

"Simplicity is the ultimate sophistication."
~ Leonardo De Vinci

E ver wonder why phone numbers are seven digits? Ask a friend to make a list of ten words or numbers. Read the list once, and then try to recall the items. Most people max out at seven or fewer. Numerous psychology experiments have found that, on average, the longest sequence the normal person can recall is about seven items.[10]

This is just one example of how the brain can only process a small amount of information at a given time. Once this threshold is surpassed, the brain's ability to cognitively grasp further information is severely diminished. The same applies to the world of selling. When too much information is presented at one time, the brain has difficulty making a buying decision.

One of the most famous experiments on the topic of choice involved an assortment of jams. Social scientists Sheena

Iyengar and Mark Lepper set up a tasting booth at an upscale restaurant in California. The first week, twenty-four different jams were available to taste. Despite many people tasting the jams, only 3 percent made a purchase. The following week, the selection was reduced to only six jams available to taste. Sales increased 900 percent![11]

Retailers, aware of how choice can impact consumer purchasing, have also explored ways to increase sales by limiting choices. One major retailer eliminated two brands of peanut butter and their peanut butter sales rose. Procter & Gamble also reduced the range of skin-care products at some of their retail outlets and sales of the products still on the shelves increased.[12]

As mentioned above, the brain can quickly become overwhelmed and confused when presented with numerous choices. The old brain, as we've referred to it, prefers simplicity over complexity. It wants assurance that it's making a good decision and the more convoluted the choosing process, the less certain it is. This leads to consumers struggling to make a decision, or if a decision is made the buyer is plagued with doubt over whether they made the right decision.

Can I help you?

When shopping for clothes, I am often approached by a salesperson asking if I need help. My typical response is

"Thanks but I'm just looking." The salesperson replies with "Ok, let me know if you need anything" and politely walks away. However; a good salesperson never wanders too far.

Staring at a wall of 200 dress shirts, I finally pick one and head to the dressing room. When I exit the dressing room to seek out a mirror, the savvy salesperson has taken the liberty of lining up a few additional shirts, laid out nicely on a table with assorted tie combinations, matching socks and a few pairs of pants. I'm no longer focused on the wall of shirts and the plethora of tie stands, I'm now interested in how I'll look in the attire laid out before me. Instead of just purchasing one shirt or maybe not making a purchase at all, I will soon be standing in front of a mirror evaluating myself in an entirely new outfit. "And by the way," says the smiling salesperson, "we're running a sale on sportscoats!"

Aside from limiting choices, some other principles mentioned in this book are at play here. When approached by a salesperson, my response is typically to decline the offer for assistance. And yet at the same time, I don't like the uncertainty that comes with having to make a purchase decision amidst numerous options. Clearly, I am leaning away from the salesperson at the onset. My old brain only sees someone who wants to sell me something. There is a trust gap that needs to be closed. Upon seeing the impressive hand-picked selection of clothing, trust grows as I now see the salesperson as competent and knowledgeable about the products he sells. Also, I am no longer engulfed in a plethora of options making it cognitively challenging to make a decision. At this point I am no longer leaning away from the salesperson, I am leaning in. This is no longer just someone trying to sell me something, it's a person with a name who is making it easy for me to get what I want.

I've heard many practice owners mention, sometimes complain, about an optician that takes a "long time" selling a pair of glasses. This usually involves someone who insists on presenting dozens of frame and lens options in a well-intended effort to make sure the patient is happy with his or her new eyewear. Some opticians prefer to let the patient independently browse the 850 frames that line the walls of your optical and pick out several that they like. Some opticians will review every lens option available along with what's covered by the patient's vision insurance. They pride themselves on thoroughness. While it's important that patients are informed and educated, how much is too much? Would fewer choices and a more streamlined approach promote better outcomes?

It's not just the optical where this is relevant. One time I was asked to review a doctor's contact lens exam fees and he sent me a spreadsheet of twelve different fees all within ten dollars of each other. One OD, in an attempt to sell more services that were not covered by the patient's vision plan, presented patients at check-in with a list of eight different add-on services and asked them to pick two. I've seen employee bonus plans so complicated I needed a financial adviser to explain it to me. With our patients, employees and even ourselves, are we sometimes making things unnecessarily complicated?

It was so simple!

A few years ago the consulting firm I work for conducted an experiment. We secret shopped a well-known online optical retailer that had recently started selling glasses out of brick and mortar stores in addition to the Internet. All of the consultants visited the store separately. I was the only consultant with an OD degree, and I found the feedback from the other non-OD consultants to be very interesting. Their experience may have been more aligned with the typical consumer. After everyone had visited the store and we met to share notes, each consultant unanimously agreed that what they liked most about the experience was how simple the process was. At the time, this retailer did not accept insurance and had two prices, one for single vision and another for progressives. No lengthy forms to complete. No complicated pricing structures. No painful explanations of insurance coverage. Nobody pecking away at a calculator to determine out of pocket costs. It was clean and simple!

I am aware that this retailer offers a different business model than the typical OD owned private practice. I am not attempting to make an apples-to-apples comparison, because, for one, we do have to deal with vision plans and a lot of other regulatory matters that make this level of simplicity nearly impossible, but the lesson was still enlightening and leads to asking if we could simplify the experience for patients in a traditional practice. Let's revisit my friend from earlier in the book who was disappointed with his eye exam. He had mentioned the wide selection of frames along with all the information he received from the doctor and staff, and yet he did not make a purchase. The problem was not a lack of information or options, the problem was his difficulty evaluating the worth of the products being sold. Too many choices and too much information, while well-intended, obstructs the brains capacity to make a decision.

The good news is that this presents a great opportunity to better serve your patients. Before you overwhelm a patient with a lengthy list of services and fees at check-in, plethora of treatment options in the exam lane, and then send them to a room filled with frames in every direction, let's consider how we can make the experience less cognitively demanding for the patient. Ask yourself if you are presenting too much information or too many choices. Is it possible you would be more successful with providing consumers with only (or mostly) the information they need to make a positive buying decision? For people in sales positions, as their knowledge about the products and services they sell increases, over time the amount of information in their presentations can increase as well. What can you cut out without sacrificing value? As the saying goes, sometimes less is more.

Messages that stick

In the book *Made to Stick: Why Some Ideas Survive and Others Die* by Chip Heath and Dan Heath, simplicity is presented as one of the core elements of an idea or message that sticks. The authors are careful to mention that simple is not about dumbing down, rather it is about prioritization. It is about trimming ideas down to what really matters. Doctors, opticians and other specialists tend to appreciate and gravitate toward complexity. Many doctors, by nature, are fascinated by nuance and complexity. This is where something referred to as the "curse of knowledge" kicks in. The curse of knowledge leads to forgetting what it's like *not* to know what we know – so we ramble on with lengthy explanations of eye pathology, lens technology, diagnostic test results, and a lot of clinical jargon peppered into the discussion. We fear that stripping down a message will devolve into oversimplification. It's more likely that what we call educating will devolve into confusion.

Ironically, as I'm typing this, a comment came across my Facebook feed from an OD mentioning a patient had complained to his staff that the doctor made him feel "terminology shamed."

Let me share an example using fruit. In *Made to Stick*, the authors share the following example of an explanation of a piece of fruit called a pomelo.[13]

EXPLANATION 1: A pomelo is the largest citrus fruit. The rind is very thick but soft and easy to peel away. The resulting fruit has a light yellow to coral pink flesh and can vary from juicy to slightly dry and from seductively spicy-sweet to tangy and tart.

Now close your eyes and try to imagine eating a pomelo. More than likely, your brain is struggling to process this mental image. Now read the next explanation and again imagine yourself eating a pomelo.

EXPLANATION 2: A pomelo is basically a supersized grapefruit with a very thick and soft rind.

If instead of choosing a career in optometry, you had chosen to become a fruitologist (I made that word up), then you might be tempted to offer the first explanation. Right, smarty pants? But as a fruit consumer, which explanation would be more likely to *stick* with you? Assuming you're hungry and you like fruit, what explanation would be more likely to lead you to make a purchase?

Since most optometrists do not sell fruit in their practice, I'll share with you some scripting we provide our consulting members. You can use this as a training resource for your staff. This was designed with the intent of being simple and memorable. As discussed, simple is not dumbing down the message, it's a process of getting to the core of the message and delivering it in a compact manner. If a patient feels confused or overwhelmed with the information they are provided, the message will not stick!

Optometry practice scripting

1. Front Desk Incoming
   a. "Thank you for calling [Practice Name] this is [name] how may I help you?
   b. Scheduling Appointments
      i. You'd like to schedule an appointment? Terrific, have you been our practice before?
         1. You have? Excellent, could I please get your name so I can look up your information? Thank you.
            a. It looks like you saw [Doctor] on [date] for a comprehensive exam does that sound about right? [Verify patient's insurance, address, contact info, etc.]
               i. Are you wearing any contact lenses right now? Do you think that's something you might be interested in?

      ii. I see here that your [family member] was also seen at that time, will you be scheduling their exam today as well?

    b. It looks like you saw [Doctor] on [date] for a contact lens exam does that sound about right? [Verify patient's insurance, address, contact info, etc.]

        i. Excellent, how are you doing with your contacts?

       ii. Your insurance shows that your [family member(s)] is/are also eligible for eye exams, will you be scheduling their exam(s) today as well?

ii. What day works best for you? Alright, a Thursday. Would you prefer [available AM slot] or [available PM slot]? Perfect, thank you so much! We'll see you on [confirm date], and make sure to bring in all your existing prescription glasses and sunglasses, thank you!

c. Insurance questions

    i. Do we take [In-Network Insurance]? Absolutely we do! We can submit everything for you right on the spot, and you're going to get a terrific discount on your exam and your glasses!

    ii. Do we take [Out of Network Insurance]? Absolutely we do! We'd be happy to fill out all your claim paperwork for you, all you have to do is mail it in, and you'll get a reimbursement check in the mail! You'll get a terrific discount on your exam and your glasses!

d. Optical Questions

    i. Could I place you on hold for just a moment? I'd like to transfer you to our Optician, [he/she] is an expert at providing you all the information about that you might need. Thank you.

2. Front Desk Outgoing/Recalls

a. This is [name] calling on behalf of [Doctor], to remind [Patient] that it's time for [his/her] annual eye exam. When can I schedule that appointment?

b. This is [name] calling on behalf of [Doctor], to confirm [Patient]'s appointment on [Pre-Appointment Date and Time]. If you have any questions, please feel free to call at [Phone Number]. We'll see you on [confirm date], and make sure to bring in all your existing prescription glasses and sunglasses, thank you!

3. Optician/Sales

    a. Discovery/Open Ended Questions – These questions open up the lines of communication between the optician and the patient. It makes the interaction less of a transaction and more of a service. The Optician asks questions and the patient shares information about themselves in a conversation that doesn't necessarily indicate that it's about glasses. Later, when the optician recalls pertinent information from the dialogue, the patient understands that the optician is recommending for the patient's individual lifestyle, rather than a blanket recommendation for all patients.

        i. **What do you do for work?** (Make note of heavy computer use or fluorescent lighting for A/R and workplace progressives, indoor/outdoor for transitions, lots of outside work for Rx sun, etc.)

        ii. **What about outside of work, what do you do for fun?** (Note outdoor activities with specialized solutions. Avid golfers (G30 lens from Oakley, Maui Rose from Maui Jim, etc.), fishing (Deep Blue Polarized from Oakley, HCL from Maui Jim, etc.), knitting, beading, jewelry making (dedicated readers or lined bifocals for finer work, etc.) and so on.

iii. **What don't you like about your current glasses?** (Note responses, durability, clarity, comfort, appearance, etc.)

iv. **What do you like about your current glasses?** (Style, fit, etc.)

v. **Anything big planned for [The summer, the holidays, the weekend, etc.]?** (Big events like weddings or parties where people will be taking pictures, talk about A/R or even contact lenses. Going on vacation? Sunglasses. Also, take this opportunity to develop your rapport with your patient. Your recommendations carry more weight when the patient likes you.

b. A/R

i. Do you want lenses with glare or without?

ii. You mentioned that you spend a lot of time working at the computer. We can make a lens for you that keeps your eyes from getting overly tired throughout the day. How does that sound?

iii. Our anti-reflective coating will help your glasses look much nicer. The coating makes your lenses almost invisible. You won't get that annoying flash on your lenses in pictures, people will be able to see your beautiful eyes and it makes your lenses appear thinner.

iv. If the patient has a high plus Rx – Your prescription is a high plus power, meaning that your lenses are magnifying lenses. So with your glasses now, you can see that your eyes look slightly larger than they actually are, with the Anti-Reflective coating, that won't happen. This helps your glasses look like a more natural accessory, one that compliments your features.

v. If the patient has a high minus Rx – Your prescription is a high minus power, meaning that your lenses are minifying lenses. So with your glasses now, you can see that your eyes look slightly smaller than they actually are, with the Anti-Reflective coating, that won't happen. This helps your glasses look like a more natural accessory, one that compliments your features.

vi. After an objection – I understand that you've never had the anti-reflective coating before, but that doesn't mean you shouldn't get it this time around. Your lenses without the coating actually reflect 8-12% of light* without the coating, that's light that's not getting to your eye, making your world a little dimmer. Imagine if you went home and turned down the brightness on your television by 12%. Of course you could see it, but it wouldn't be nearly as sharp as it could or should be!

c. Progressive Types

    i. Progressive lenses allow you to see far away (for driving, watching television and movies) up close (reading, knitting, fine work) and at every distance in between. Lined or traditional bifocals have your distance correction, your reading correction, and that's it. Progressives allow you to wear one pair of glasses for most of your day to day activities.

    ii. Progressive lenses usually have a bit of an adjustment period when you first get them, especially if you've worn lined bifocals in the past. We want you to wear your new progressives full time for at least two weeks to make certain you've adapted to them.

    iii. There are many different brands or types of progressives, many of which serve different purposes. You mentioned to me that you like to read, so we want to provide you a progressive that has a wide and sharp reading channel to minimize how much you have to move your head to read clearly.

iv. We recommend [Lens of Choice] because it has the best technology for you. It's a digital or free form progressive lens. What that means is that it's a lens that is tailor made for your prescription, for the frame that you chose, and for the measurements that I've taken/will take.

1. Progressives generally come from large blank lenses with the progressive design already built in to it. Your prescription would then be ground into the blank, and then the lens would be cut out of that blank to fit your frame.

2. With a digital lens, there is no design until our lab has all the information it needs. The design is then digitally applied to the lens blank, allowing for the clearest, most natural vision we can provide.

d. Transitions

i. Regular

1. Transitions lenses will darken whenever you go outside, and will get darkest in cold weather. They're an

incredibly versatile lens that makes it easy to go from indoors to outdoors without having to switch glasses.

2. Patient says, "So if I get transitions, I don't need sunglasses, right?"

    a. You should know that these lenses don't replace prescription sunglasses for a number of reasons. First, they're not polarized. And second, transition lenses react to ultraviolet light, that's how they turn dark; when you're in the car, the windshield filters out UV light, so that it never hits your lenses. If UV light doesn't hit your lenses, they don't darken.

3. Patient says, "Will they look dark when I'm inside?"

    a. When you first get your transitions lenses, they'll be perfectly clear indoors and darken when you go out. The longer you wear them though, the more of a residual tint your lenses will have even when you're indoors. It won't impact how you see out of them, but people will be able to see the tint after about 8 months or so.

4. "Will they get dark when I'm using a computer?"

    a. No, they won't darken when you're using a computer, they react to ultraviolet light.

5. Patient says, "I've had transitions before, and they take too long to turn."

    a. Transitions have been around for a while now, and they're on their seventh generation of lenses. They now get darker than ever before, more quickly than ever before. It takes about 30 seconds for them to get as dark as they can, and about 75 seconds for them to clear again when you return indoors.

    ii. Vantage

        1. Transitions Vantage lenses have a lot of the same properties as regular transitions lenses with one major advantage. Variable Polarization. What that means is that when you go outside, your lenses become just like polarized sunglasses, isn't that amazing?

            a. You should know though, they start out a little bit darker than regular transitions do, here, let me show you an example of what they'll look like.

            b. Like transitions, they won't darken when you're inside a car, so for driving you'll still want prescription sunglasses.

    iii. Xtra Active

        1. These lenses start out darker than traditional transitions and they **will** darken when you're driving, but they're not polarized. A great option for people who are in and out of their cars all day.

    iv. Drivewear

        1. Drivewear lenses are polarized and start with a mild orange tint when indoors and they react to both visible and ultraviolet light. When driving, they get slightly darker, and when outside they get darker still. A great option for sunglasses that react to changing light conditions.

  e. Polarization

    i. Polarization is when a sunglass lens filters light in a very specific way. Without a polarizing filter, light comes into your eyes from all directions, but when polarized, it only comes in from one direction, like a pole. The result is a clearer, sharper, more vibrant world with less squinting and strain for you.

    ii. Polarized sunglasses eliminate blinding sun glare off of reflective surfaces like windshields, bumpers, water, and snow. They also help you see through some reflective surfaces more clearly, making them ideal for driving or fishing.

    iii. Gray Polarized

        1. Gray Polarized lenses are great for very sunny days, and they allow for

true colors to shine through while keeping your eyes comfortable.

    iv. Brown Polarized

        1. Brown Polarized lenses are a terrific all-purpose sunglass lens. They increase contrasts, improving your depth perception. These lenses reduce blue light transmission and are great for varying sun conditions. (Overcast to sunny and back again.)

f. Blue Light Lenses

    i. Lenses that are designed to protect your eyes from high energy blue light are very important in our modern-day life. You say you spend time working on a computer and/or under fluorescent lights, even looking at your cell phone or tablet exposes your eyes to blue light. These lenses were built from the ground up to defend your eyes from the dangers of blue light and to keep your eyes and your vision healthy.

g. Frames

h. 2nd pair benefits – Here, we want to tie the information we learned from the patient during our discovery with their need for not just two pairs of glasses, but sometimes three or four.

i. "Mr. Jones, you've told me that you work on a computer for at least eight hours a day, you watch TV in bed every night and you like to golf on the weekends, does that sound right? Perfect. So let's find you some glasses to take care of all of your visual needs.

Possibilities:

1. Workplace Progressives
2. Distance only a/r coated lenses
3. Polarized sunglasses
4. All purpose progressives
5. Progressive Sunglasses.

[Obviously, most patients won't be buying 5 pairs of glasses, but we want patients to know that there are solutions for all their visual needs, and that we want nothing more than to provide them.]

i. Recap

i. So we've got your everyday glasses, the lenses will be thin, light, non-glare, and the progressive will get you the clearest vision possible. Your sunglasses are going to be gray polarized lenses with the backside AR coating, so that you can go fishing and not be bothered by the reflections off the water. Your reading glasses are also going to be non-glare, and they'll make it so you can read without having to move your head at all like in your progressives. Does that all sound right?

4. Insurance Benefits

a. Do we take [In-Network Insurance]? Absolutely we do! We can submit everything for you right on the spot, and you're going to get a terrific discount on your exam and your glasses!

i. It looks like you'll get a discount of [Frame allowance] on your frames and some really great discounts on your lenses for your first pair of glasses. Also, you've got a significant discount for each additional pair of glasses, so we can get you those sunglasses you talked about with the doctor.

b. Do we take [Out of Network Insurance]? Absolutely we do! We'd be happy to fill out all your claim paperwork for you, all you have to do is mail it in, and you'll get a reimbursement check in the mail! You'll get a terrific discount on your exam and your glasses!

i. It looks like you'll get a discount of [Frame allowance] on your frames and some really great discounts on your lenses for your first pair of glasses. Also, you've got a significant discount for each additional pair of glasses, so we can get you those sunglasses you talked about with the doctor.

5. Contact Lenses
   a. Year Supply pricing/rebates
      i. I see the doctor has prescribed [Contact Lenses] for you, that's great!
   b. Daily Disposable Benefits
   c. Compliance
   d. I & R Training
6. Remakes/Recovery
7. Optometrist Transition to Optical

CHAPTER SEVEN:

Unlock the Language of the Subconscious Mind

"Language is the light of the mind."

~ John Stuart Mill

Throughout much of this book we've referred to the subconscious brain, or "old brain", as the true decision maker. That being the case, it will benefit you and your staff greatly to learn the language of the subconscious mind. As it turns out, the decision-making part of the brain responds to a set of very specific stimuli. Introducing these stimuli into your conversations and presentations will greatly enhance your ability to persuade and influence.

In the book *Neuromarketing: Understanding the Buy Buttons in Your Customer's Brain*, author and researcher Patrick Renvoise identified the only six stimuli that speak to the old brain. Imagine if English is the only language you understand, and somebody approached you speaking French. Obviously, the message will not get through to the receiver. But as soon as this person begins speaking

English, you are suddenly able to process the information. It bears repeating that a very specific part of the brain is responsible for most of our decisions and if we want to more effectively communicate with that part of the brain, we have to speak its language! Below are the six stimuli that have been scientifically proven to make your recommendations and ideas more impactful.[14]

#1 Self-centered

The old brain is very narcissistic. Allow me to use *my* old brain as an example.

Upon graduating from optometry school, I decided to treat myself to a massive purchase – shoes! Exciting, huh? Like many new grads, I didn't have much money when I came out of school, but I sure owed a lot! Nonetheless, I decided to treat myself to a nice pair of dress shoes from Nordstrom, a rather high-end retailer. I recall paying around $150 for the shoes, which at that point in my life was a serious outlay of cash.

Fast forward six months, and a slight problem developed with this grand purchase of mine. The soles of the shoes began coming off! They were unwearable. While disappointed, I had for the most part always operated under the *caveat emptor* policy, otherwise known as "buyer beware." However; this particular time I decided to take a stand. For what I paid, I really felt this purchase should have lasted longer than six months. So I grabbed the shoes, hopped in the car, and headed to Nordstrom.

Walking into the store, I admit to being a bit reluctant. A part of me felt that I was being unreasonable, after all, I had owned the shoes for nearly half a year. Truthfully, I expected to hear about the store's return policy, perhaps be told I needed to speak with a manager, and then likely be denied in my request for reconciliation. But this was a matter of principle! The little guy standing up to the big corporation! I wanted them to know of my disappointment, and maybe they would throw me a bone like a coupon or discount on my next purchase.

As I walked through the door, I immediately spotted a salesperson and walked right up to him. I had even rehearsed my story on the car ride over, prepared for someone to give me an annoyed look and recite the company's return policy. To my surprise, that's not what I received. About 90 seconds into my speech, the salesperson had all the information he needed. He then snatched the shoes out of my hands, said he would be right back, and walked away. Not quite sure how to interpret that, I waited patiently for his return. A few moments later the salesperson returned carrying a brand-new pair of shoes, handed them to me with a smile, and asked if there was anything else he could do for me.

Me, Me, Me!

I love ODs. I think it's a wonderful profession made up of great people. I've had the pleasure of meeting many great eye care professionals who genuinely care about the patients they treat and the employees they provide jobs for. Many go above and beyond to serve their patients and their community, and many are involved with efforts of giving back outside of their practice. It's a wonderful group of people, and yet, as *consumers* we all become the person I described who returned a six-month old pair of shoes – we become self-centered!

I have to be honest. When I walked into Nordstrom I wasn't concerned at all about the company. I didn't want to hear about any return policies or restocking fees. I didn't care if this created extra work for a company employee. I didn't care if the company was losing money in this transaction. All I cared about was me! I paid a lot of money for shoes that were no longer functional. What are you going to do for ME?

As consumers, this is the question we are always asking. How does this benefit me? How will this solve a problem for me? What can you do for me?

As a reminder, this does not mean we are all selfish, greedy jerks. Qualities like compassion and empathy are evident in most people, but in regard to decision making –

including purchase decisions – we are operating from a different part of the brain. The next patient who walks through your door may very well love puppy dogs, send flowers to his mom every Mother's Day and do volunteer work in under-privileged neighborhoods, but as an eyewear consumer he is mostly just interested in how your products and services will benefit him. This is the old brain at work, and the old brain has no patience or empathy for things that do not concern its well-being and survival.

You, You, You!

Now that we better understand the narcissistic nature of the consumer mind, let's consider two competing approaches optometry practices can take with patients. Below are comments I frequently hear from doctors and their staff.

If patients aren't willing to abide by MY policies…

If people aren't willing to conform to MY rules…

If they don't respect MY time… then they can go somewhere else!

Can you see the conflict this creates between the business and the consumer? Business owners often want it both ways. As consumers, they want the places they conduct business with to bend over backwards to meet their needs, even if it means bending the rules. As business / practice owners, they want the consumer to conform to the policies and preferences of the practice. Both sides are pointing at themselves saying "Me, Me, Me!" For many practice owners, there's a good chance if you could somehow clone yourself and the consumer version of you walked into your practice, the two of you would not get along. It might end with you kicking yourself out of your practice and then consumer you writing a bad review… about You!

There's a reason that Nordstrom is a $15 billion company, my story is just one small example. Nordstrom, along with most other great companies that rise to the top through great customer service, understands this one simple thing that separates it from competitors that struggle to grow and compete. Regardless of what you sell, in any service-based industry the top performers understand the mind of the consumer and instead of insisting "Me, Me, Me!", these companies build a culture of "You, You, You!" In other words, they are aligning their business model and selling strategies with what's important to the consumer. To quote a mentor of mine, Dr. Neil Gailmard, "Let the patient win!"

To revisit a concept discussed earlier, as a consumer what happens when you sense that an individual or company you are doing business with is putting their interests above yours? You being to lean away! It's very difficult to sell anyone a product, service or idea when they are leaning away. Leaning away indicates a lack of trust.

I am not suggesting you always side with the patient or acquiesce to their demands. I've heard the common objections to a You culture many, many times.

We can't let the patients walk all over us!

The patient is being unreasonable!

We need to stand our ground!

Granted there are times when you have to take a stand. Even Disney World, world renowned for its legendary customer service, sometimes has to deny a request or tell a patron they are no longer welcome at their theme park. However; that is the rare exception. If you want to run a business with a "Me, Me, Me!" mentality, you can certainly do that. It's your practice. Just know that from a consumer psychology standpoint you will often be at odds with the very people who purchase from you – your patients!

A lot of practice owners lose sleep over the success of their business, implementing a lot of policies and rules to protect their interests. If you're willing to try a different approach, you might discover what a lot of successful business owners already know. If instead of losing so much sleep over the success of your business you spent more time losing sleep over the success of your patient, you would probably end up losing a lot less sleep.

"The customer is always right" is not a fact, it's a business strategy.

#2 Visuals

Years ago, a patient of mine who happened to be a good friend presented for his yearly eye exam. This particular patient had a history of not being fully compliant with my recommendations to remove his contact lenses at night. He had been developing corneal neovascularization that appeared to worsen at each visit. Seeing that the condition had once again worsened, I gave him very stern instructions. "As your eye care professional, it's incumbent upon me to inform you that sleeping in your contact lenses is resulting in corneal oxygen deprivation and as a response the body is attempting to provide necessary nutrients and oxygen to the deprived corneal tissues by creating new blood vessels. If this blood vessel encroachment continues, this can cause a variety of symptoms including tearing, light sensitivity, redness, scarring and decreased vision." Actually, because this was a close friend of mine the conversation went more like this, "Dude, take your damn contacts out at night!"

History told me my pleas for him to take this more seriously would get a genuine, "Yeah, I know, I promise I'll try harder!" And he would for a short time, and then old habits would eventually resume. For whatever reasons, verbal explanations never had a strong impact on getting my friend to change his behavior. In other words, I wasn't very persuasive. So I decided to try something new. As he was giving me his yearly "I'll try harder" speech, I pulled up a picture of corneal neovascularization on my computer and pointed at it. His reaction was strong and immediate. He glanced at the picture and almost immediately turned away saying, "Ugh, that's what's happening to my eyes! That looks awful!" He literally begged me to close out the picture and promised me he would regularly remove the contact lenses at night, which he made a point of telling me periodically that since seeing that picture he made sure to remove the contacts every night. This was a real "a-ha" moment for me in terms of getting a point across. Use visuals!

I have an image I use in one of my presentations of the Michelin baby sitting next to a tire with the caption, "MICHELIN, BECAUSE SO MUCH IS RIDING ON YOUR TIRES." The baby and tire are centered in the picture and take up much of the space. In the lower right corner there are a few small paragraphs of text in very small print size. I have yet to actually read the paragraphs. The company's marketing department took the time to include this in the ad, so I'm sure in some capacity the information is important. Nevertheless, I suspect that Michelin is not too concerned whether or not you read the text. What do they want you to remember? The baby sitting next to the tire!

The old brain is visual. It responds faster to visual images and retains visuals much longer than written or verbal communication. Anatomically, the optic nerve is physically connected to the old brain and processes information 25 times faster than the auditory nerve.[14] Some studies have found that people forget much of what they hear within 24 hours when not accompanied with visual imagery.

The reality is that the old brain is not very smart. The newer parts of the brain like the outer cortex is adept at processing words, ideas and concepts, but the old brain doesn't speak that language. While it is certainly necessary to provide patients with written and verbal information that is relevant to the care of their eyes, whenever possible use visuals to enhance the patient's level of understanding. The visual channel provides a fast and effective connection to the true decision-maker.

#3 Emotion

In one of my presentations titled The Science of Selling, I tell the audience that I am going to show them a commercial for a car manufacturer. I set up the video by offering a challenge. I tell the audience that every time they hear some sort of technical feature about the car, like an engineering feature or safety function, to write it down on the pad of paper in front of them and at the end of the commercial we will see who has the longest list. I mention they will have to write quickly because the car company has to cram a lot of information into a 60 second ad. Everyone picks up a pen and gets ready to start scribbling furiously. I then hit play on the video.

The video actually portrays a young girl and her dog through different phases of life such as learning to drive, going through a breakup with a boyfriend, and going off to college – her furry friend (and a Chevy) by her side every step of the way. The video ends with the young girl, now a grown woman, kissing the nose of her now older dog and the words "A best friend for life's journey" appear as the commercial fades out. It's a heart tugging commercial, and every time I show the video I see people in the audience wiping away tears. There is no mention of any technical functions or features in this commercial. None. At the end of the commercial everyone in the audience is staring at a blank sheet of paper.

Do you think a 60 second car ad that focused on braking systems, Bluetooth capability and trunk space would have gotten this reaction? Would it have been as memorable? Consider this in your own marketing and communication efforts. I review a lot of websites as a consultant. I'm not a designer or website expert, but I do like to see a practice's website before consulting with the practice for the first time. What I find with a lot of doctor websites is they can be very clinical and feature oriented. Lengthy paragraphs about the doctor's accomplishments and background. Lists of every frame the practice carries and what insurance plans they accept. Home pages devoted to all the diagnostic technology the office has. It's a lot of "stuff", but often fails to connect with the viewer on an emotional level. Below are just a few ideas for adding more emotion to your persuasion arsenal:

- Abandon the stock images on your website and use actual pictures of your office and staff.
- Recorded patient testimonials can be powerful and memorable.
- Story telling can be a very effective emotional tool. It's why you watch movies. Tell stories of patients of yours who have experienced positive outcomes. No names of course!
- Hire a videographer to create a short practice profile video highlighting your wonderful office and friendly staff.
- Sponsor local charities or get involved with efforts to give back to your community and highlight this in your practice newsletter.
- Post fun pics on your practice Facebook page (office parties, employees dressed up for Halloween, etc.)
- Focus on building relationships with your patients. Are you in the "glasses and contact lens" business, or the "serving people" business? There's a difference.

The old brain is strongly triggered by emotion. It impacts both how we process and retain information. Science and research have found that the "chemical cocktail" produced in the brain after we experience emotion greatly enhances our memory of events and information.

As the famous quote by Maya Angelou goes, "People will forget what you said, people will forget what you did, but people will never forget how you made them feel."

#4 Contrast

As we've discussed, the decision-making part of the brain likes to make quick, risk-free decisions. As opposed to having to conduct a deep logical analysis of alternative options which can quickly confuse the old brain, contrast such as before/after, risky/safe, with/without and slow/fast provides a mechanism for faster, safer decisions.

Let me ask you this. What's the most powerful part of a weight loss ad? What grabs your attention when you're flipping through a magazine or surfing the Internet and see "Lose 30 pounds in 30 days!"? Is it the paragraphs of research that went into developing this supplement? Is it the science behind the claims or the ingredient quality? Is it the company reputation? Not to suggest these things don't matter, but what usually grabs your attention with weight loss ads? It's the before and after picture!

We've talked a lot about neuropsychology and its involvement in decision-making, and I'll continue that here. The old brain has difficulty thinking in terms of past and future.[14] Remember, this is an older, more primitive part of the brain concerned with survival and well-being. In many ways it is an animalistic part of the brain. As I'm typing this my dog Addie is sitting at my feet. She's not regretting the shoe she ate yesterday, and she's not worried about where she will get her next meal. She's only concerned with right now. That's how the old brain works. Don't tell me how much better things will be in the future if I purchase XYZ options, show me now! Contrast is a powerful tool because it allows us to bring past and future into the present moment.

In many ways, eye care providers already use contrast to demonstrate change. This could be flipping from habitual to updated Rx on a digital phoropter, dipping trial lenses over a distance Rx to demonstrate a near Rx, holding up two lenses to demonstrate with and without anti-reflective coating, or showing a patient an image of a normal fundus next to an image of diabetic retinopathy. I know of practices that have purchased cheap, low-quality frames from online vendors so patients can compare to higher quality materials. Using contrast allows people to overcome their own objections, which as you recall is the #1 enemy to making a sale. You have actually altered the consumer's perception of the facts, and yet the facts have not changed at all.

As we've already learned, the visuals themselves are powerful. Whenever it applies, introduce contrast into your discussions, presentations and marketing. Companies use these strategies all the time in comparing their offerings to their competitors. Lower prices, faster service, better quality, etc. If you told me your practice specialized in dry eye and offered patient hours on the weekend, that would be nice to know but not necessarily convert me into a patient. Once you tell me that you're the only practice in town that specializes in dry eye (a condition I struggle with) and offers weekend coverage (I work and travel a lot during the week) then you've introduced contrast. Not only does this grab the attention of my old brain, but it also allows me to feel justified in my decision to choose you as my eye care provider.

#5 Tangible

In 2009, researchers in the United Kingdom examined the impact of contact lens application in non-contact lens wearers prior to spectacle dispensing. In what was called the EASE (Enhanced Approach to Selecting Eyewear) Study, subjects were randomly placed in a test group or a control group. Both groups had no previous contact lens experience. The test group subjects were offered trial contact lenses prior to spectacle dispensing. The control subjects proceeded to spectacle dispensing without the offer to try contact lenses. At a follow-up appointment, the test group who had the opportunity to experience having contact lenses on their eyes were 3 times more likely to purchase contact lenses. Of the test group, 33% ordered contact lenses where only 13% of the control group ordered. As a side benefit, this group also spent 32% more on eyeglasses.[16]

Ever wonder why companies are so eager to offer free trials and free samples? People rarely just look at clothing and make a purchase. They want to try the clothes on! What about the people in shopping mall food courts chasing you around with a piece of teriyaki chicken on a toothpick! When you're at a car dealership looking for a new automobile, what's one of the first things you want to do when a particular automobile catches your eye? Sure, factors such as price, features and safety matter – but what do you *really* want to do before getting to all of that? You want to take it for a test drive! You want to get your hands on the steering wheel, feel the leather seats, smell that unmistakable "new car" small. Right?

One of the challenges with online retailers is they lose the advantage of tangibility when the consumer is not able to physically see, touch or experience the product in the same way they can in a brick and mortar store. This is why many online vendors have started sending the product to the consumer's home to try out before making a purchase. We are seeing this trend in the clothing and fashion industry and even some online frame vendors are now offering to send a small shipment of frames to the person's home to try on before deciding on a purchase. And if you don't like any, just send them all back. It's a wonderful strategy that reduces or even eliminates that pesky obstacle to a sale called "risk."

From a consumer psychology standpoint, tangibility is very important to the purchase. The old brain is not swayed by claims, it wants proof! Proof trumps claims every time. Don't tell me how great this car handles corners, let me see for myself! Don't tell me I'll sleep better taking this supplement, let me see for myself! Don't tell me how comfortable these contact lenses will be and how much better I will see with them, let me SEE for myself!

The old brain likes to see, feel and touch. This provides tangible proof that what you're telling me is accurate. It gets the consumer to go from leaning away to leaning in. So make sure patients, even those on the fence about a purchase, are being directed to browse your optical. In many practices, too many patients walk out without having tried on a single pair of glasses. Consider a less rigid approach to fitting contact lenses. Would sales improve if you encouraged more patients to try contact lenses at no risk and you or a tech quickly inserted a pair before the patients heads to the optical? Giving away free services you say? No way! If the patient falls in love with the idea of clear vision without glasses, we'll schedule a full CL fitting/training and charge accordingly.

What additional ways could you add more tangibility to the patient experience?

#6 Beginning and end

The old brain is more likely to remember the beginning and end of events and forget everything in between. Think of some of your favorite movies. You are more likely to vividly recall things that happened at the beginning and end of the movie, while the details in between are less memorable. If you're a music fan and got to see one of your favorite bands or performers live in concert, there's a good chance you can recall what song they opened with and also what song they closed out their encore with, but you're probably less certain about other songs played during the show. In fact, you may not even recall *if* certain songs were played even though you were at the concert.

This same principle can be applied to the patient experience. Not to say you shouldn't strive to deliver a great experience throughout the entire visit, but when the patient later thinks back to their experience in your office, first and last impressions will likely be more memorable that many of the details that occurred in between. However; for many practices the first impression involves completing a lot of paperwork including reading and signing forms detailing what will happen if you don't pay your bill or you bounce a check, and the last impression is an employee pecking away at a calculator to see how much money you owe. Yes, paperwork and fees are part of the process, but I do think there are ways to make the experience more pleasant for the patient. Or at least less painful! For example, make sure every patient who walks in the door is greeted with a wide smile and friendly introduction. "Hi Ms. Smith. I'm Kim, welcome to our office!" First impressions are so important for the old brain and can play a major factor in the patient's decision-making process throughout the rest of the visit. This can truly be a make or break moment. How much paperwork do you ask patients to complete at check-in? Nobody likes paperwork! Could you minimize it? Could you get it down to one or two forms or even have a tech do most of it during pre-testing by entering it directly into the EHR? Could you improve office efficiency so patients do not have to wait as long, or just invite them to browse the optical instead of sitting in a waiting area? Does the check-out process feel like a "transaction" for the patient, or does it feel like they are leaving a good friend's house who truly appreciated the visit?

Beginning and end can obviously involve the start and finish of the entire visit, but it can also pertain to individual encounters. If you are a doctor, consider the impression you make at the beginning and end of the exam process. How do *you* feel when you go to the doctor and a lab coat walks through the door appearing cold and unfriendly?

Hello, I'm Dr. Serious. What brings you in today?

There's a reason doctors who are friendly, humorous and engaging are much less likely to be sued than their counterparts.[15] Consider the first and last impression that you create for each patient and talk with your staff about their patient interactions as well. When we combine the "beginning and end" principle with likeability, this can be a very powerful persuasion strategy.

Again, if the next patient who walks into your practice is greeted by a distracted, unfriendly receptionist who's on a phone call and looks up just long enough to hand the patient a stack of paperwork and motions for him or her to have a seat in the waiting area, it's possible that nothing else your practice does beyond this will make much of a difference. The patient is leaning away.

Conclusion

But I don't sell.

If it wasn't obvious, the title of this book reflects the aversion many doctors and health care professionals have to the topic of selling. I hope this book helped reframe the issue for you. In a rapidly changing industry, the ability to sell your products, services and even yourself is no longer a luxury, it is a necessity! If you don't like the results you're getting, try something different. As the famous saying goes, "The definition of insanity is doing the same thing over and over and expecting different results."

This book was obviously written from the perspective of an OD, but the principles can apply to everyone in your practice. In some ways, each member of your team has a role in selling. As we've discussed throughout this book, selling can be broken down into the simplest of components such as a welcoming smile from a receptionist, an inquiry about occupation or hobbies from a tech, or a streamlined eyeglass presentation from an optician that targets the patient's unique vision needs. I think this book might be especially valuable to associate ODs. One of the most common questions I hear surrounds associate or employed ODs and their production.

"My associate does not produce as much as me."

"His revenue per patient is much lower than mine."

"A lot of her patients are walking out with their script."

These can be delicate conversations, as many non-owner ODs perceive their value to the practice as strictly clinical. "I'm a doctor, I don't sell." Conversations with associate ODs are often met with resistance or half-hearted agreements to "try harder." Sometimes owner ODs avoid these conversations altogether, quietly wishing for better production out of their associate.

To any non-owner OD reading this, I don't mean for that to sound negative or harsh. Owner ODs need to understand that your primary job *is* to provide great patient care. However; non-owner ODs would be well-suited to also understand that to be able to provide this high-level patient care, everyone must be mindful of the business as well. It's the revenues and profits that get reinvested back into the practice in the form of new technology, facility, equipment, staff, staff training, and a host of other investments that enhance both clinical care and the patient experience. You can't separate these two. Frankly, I want *my* doctor to be successful so he or she can provide me with the best staff, diagnostic technology and patient experience possible. If the primary concern of your staff is saving the patient money, you are shooting yourself in the foot. It's not our role, and in fact it's a complete disservice, for us to decide how the patient spends their money. Not only does this mentality lead to that patient not getting the best care, it ultimately leads to ALL your patients not getting the best care.

I once consulted a doctor with an anemically low average revenue per patient. When I inquired about this, he insisted that he was not going to be "pushy" with recommending products to his patients. I agree with that. Being pushy is a poor sales strategy and will likely do more harm than good. While well-intended, I think this is the crux of the problem in our industry. The perception that selling has to be pushy. It doesn't! And quite frankly, if you want to be successful with selling, it can't be! People lean away from a pushy salesperson.

As stated above, I hope the strategies taught in this book help reframe the perception of selling for you and your staff. I hope it helps overcome the aversion to selling. The point of this book was to understand your patients and serve them better. If applied, I do believe these strategies can lead to better marketing, more impactful communication and happier patients.

If you want to be more persuasive with selling or anything else that requires you to influence someone to take a desirable action, then try some of the ideas presented in this book. Ask more questions and do more listening. Tap into people's emotions. Address people's objections and earn their trust. Be friendly and likeable. Do more giving than taking. Make the experience more enjoyable for the patient and less mundane and transactional. Educate without alienating and confusing. Get out of the glasses and contact lens business and get into the "serving people" business!

When you look at it this way, "selling" doesn't sound so bad, does it?

References

1. Lynette Ryals and Iain Davies. "Do You Really Know Who Your Best Salespeople Are?" *Harvard Business Review*, https://hbr.org/2010/12/vision-statement-do-you-really-know-who-your-best-salespeople-are

2. Antonio Damasio. *Descartes' Error: Emotion, Reason, and the Human Brain*. New York: Penguin Books, 2005, 193–94.

3. David Hoffeld. *The Science of Selling: Proven Strategies to Make Your Pitch, Influence Decisions, and Close the Deal*. Penguin Publishing Group.

4. Brandon Keim. "Brain Scanners Can See Your Decisions Before You Make Them." Wired, https://www.wired.com/2008/04/mind-decision/

5. Robert Cialdini. *Influence: The Psychology of Persuasion*. Harper Business, 2006.

6. William Grimes. "In War Against No-Shows, Restaurants Get Tougher." New York Times, October 15, 1997, www.nytimes.com/1997/10/15/dining/in-war-against-no-shows-restaurants-get-tougher.html?pagewanted=all.

7. Amy J. C. Cuddy, Matthew Kohut, and John Neffinger. "Connect, Then Lead." *Harvard Business Review* (July–August 2013): 56.

8. D. B. Strohmetz, B. Rind, R. Fisher, and M. Lynn. "Sweetening the Till: The Use of Candy to Increase Restaurant Tipping." *Journal of Applied Social Psychology* 32 (2002): 300–9; D. Kenny and W. Nasby. "Splitting the Reciprocity Correlations." *Journal of Personality and Social Psychology* 38 (1980): 439–48.

9. Kay-Yut Chen and Marina Krakovsky. *Secrets of the Moneylab: How Behavioral Economics Can Improve Your Business* (New York: Portfolio/Penguin, 2010); M. Morris, J. Nadler, T. Kurtzberg, and L. Thompson. "Schmooze or Lose: Social Friction and Lubrication in Email Negotiations." *Group Dynamics* 6 (2002): 89–100.

10. Lauren Schenkman. "In the Brain, Seven Is A Magic Number." ABC News, https://abcnews.go.com/Technology/brain-memory-magic-number/story?id=9189664

11. Sheena S. Iyengar and Mark R. Lepper. "When Choice Is Demotivating: Can One Desire Too Much of a Good Thing." *Journal of Personality and Social Psychology* 79 (2000): 995–1006.

12. Marina Strauss. "In Store Aisles, Less Is More but Customers Can Still Be Particular." *Globe and Mail,* May 18, 2010.

13. Chip Heath. *Made to Stick: Why Some Ideas Survive and Others Die.* Random House Publishing Group, 2007.

14. Patrick Renvoick. *Neuromarketing: Understanding the Buy Buttons in Your Customer's Brain.* Harper Collins Leadership, 2007.

15. Tamara Shopsin. "To Be Sued Less, Doctors Should Consider Talking to Patients More." The New York Times, https://www.nytimes.com/2015/06/02/upshot/to-be-sued-less-doctors-should-talk-to-patients-more.html

16. Nick Atkins, Sarah Morgan, Phillip Morgan. "Enhancing the approach to selecting eyewear (EASE): A multi-centre, practice-based study into the effect of applying contact lenses prior to spectacle dispensing." *Contact Lens and Anterior Eye.* Volume 32, Issue 3, June 2009, pages 103-107

17. Roger Dooley. *Brainfluence: 100 Ways to Persuade and Influence Consumers with Neuromarketing.* Wiley, 2011.

About the Author

Steve Vargo, OD, MBA is a 1998 graduate of the Illinois College of Optometry. In 2014 he joined Prima Eye Group (now IDOC) as Vice President of Optometric Consulting. A published author and speaker with 15 years of clinical experience, he now serves as IDOC's Optometric Practice Management Consultant. Since transitioning to a full-time practice management consultant, Dr. Vargo has performed over 3,000 consultations and coaching sessions with hundreds of independent optometry practices across the country. He speaks regularly at industry conferences, has been published in numerous industry publications, has a regular column in Optometric Management titled "The CEO Checklist", and is a contributing author to the widely read "Optometric Management Tip of the Week" article. Dr. Vargo has also authored 2 books on the subjects of staff management and leadership.

Dr. Vargo's other books (both available on Amazon):

Eye on Management: Step-by-step guide to optometry's most common staff management challenges

Eye on Leadership: An optometrist's game plan for creating a motivated and empowered team

Questions or Comments?

I'd love to hear your thoughts. Email me at: Svargo@idoc.net.

NEED HELP?

I offer consulting services to independent eye care practices through IDOC. I'll help you transform your staff and your practice. Learn more at www.IDOC.net.

54504043R00086

Made in the USA
Columbia, SC
01 April 2019